CPC Study Guide

Unlock Your Medical Coding Career With The Ultimate Step-by-Step Success Strategy | Expert Tips to Master the Test and Get Certified | Over 300 Practice Questions Included

Rusty Regent

Table of Contents

Introduction

What is the CPC Exam?

The Certified Professional Coder (CPC) credential is a certification that demonstrates a candidate's command of the diagnoses, procedures, and reimbursement standards that are essential to the administration of modern healthcare. Over the course of five hours of rigorous examination, multiple choice questions examine the candidate's grasp of anatomy, nomenclature, CPT, ICD, and HCPCS. Acquiring this certificate is not easy, but doing so demonstrates a dedication to coding accuracy, which in turn protects patients via lawful billing practices.

In addition to the consequences on one's job, successfully completing the CPC generates interest for coding. The process of deciphering medical paperwork puts one in the position of the patient being described, which improves both understanding and empathy. In a similar manner, connecting codes sheds light on a tale contained within each record, which is how therapy enhances people's lives. Because of this training, coders are able to sense the meaning behind a diagnosis rather than relying just on alphanumeric.

Self-care is an essential component of CPC preparation, in addition to academic work. Learning is most effective in minds that have been well-rested and fed. If you feel your stress level rising, take a moment to stop and reflect on the beauty that can be discovered even in the most difficult of life's chapters. In a similar vein, make use of timetables that are organized yet flexible, bringing together your career, your study, and your free time. Not the harsh tempo of perfectionism, but consistent, self-compassionate labor is what leads to forward movement.

Benefits of Becoming a Certified Professional Coder

Obtaining certification as a Certified Professional Coder (CPC) offers several opportunities for professional growth within the ever-evolving healthcare industry. This certification serves to validate one's proficiency in the domain of medical coding, while also establishing one's worth as a significant resource for healthcare companies. Healthcare corporations consistently seek competent personnel who can contribute to the enhancement of their enterprises. The subsequent enumeration is a compilation of the foremost benefits associated with obtaining a Certified Professional Coder (CPC) credential.

The prospects for a professional vocation and assured job placement

The healthcare sector is seeing continuous growth, leading to a heightened need for proficient medical coders. Possessing a Certified Professional Coder (CPC) credential might confer a competitive edge to job seekers in the current employment landscape. Healthcare providers, including hospitals, clinics, insurance companies, and other entities in the healthcare industry, have a significant need for certified professionals who possess the expertise to navigate the intricacies of medical coding. After obtaining this certification, individuals may choose to follow several career routes such as medical coding, coding specialization, medical records coordination, or billing specialization. Furthermore, it is worth noting that there exists a perpetual need for medical services, hence guaranteeing a continuous availability of employment opportunities within this particular industry.

There exists the potential for heightened financial profitability.

On the general, Certified Professional Coders (CPCs) tend to earn higher incomes compared to their non-credentialed counterparts. According to the findings of the annual salary study carried out by the AAPC, it has been observed that qualified coders tend to receive around 20% more remuneration compared to their non-certified counterparts. The discrepancy in salary can be attributed to the distinct set of abilities and expertise that a Certified Professional Coder (CPC) possesses. CPC is an acronym that denotes the professional designation of certified pharmacy technician. The possibility for your salary to increase further is contingent upon acquiring further expertise and certificates within the respective sector.

The importance of credibility and acknowledgment in the professional realm cannot be overstated. These two factors play a significant role in establishing one's reputation and success in their chosen field. Credibility refers to the level of trust and confidence that others have in an individual's knowledge, expertise, and abilities. It is built over time by consistent

Obtaining the Certified Professional Coder (CPC) certification serves as evidence to prospective employers, colleagues, and patients that one possesses the requisite competencies and professionalism essential for fulfilling the rigorous demands of the healthcare industry. This demonstrates the individual's commitment to their career and their competence in adhering to rigorous coding protocols. This professional recognition has the ability to enhance your credibility and increase the opportunities for career advancement.

Continual Acquisition of Knowledge and Skill Enhancement
The field of medical coding is characterized by its continuous evolution, since coding rules and standards are often updated to include the latest breakthroughs in medical knowledge and technology. The acquisition of Continuing Education Units (CEUs) through ongoing study is vital for maintaining the currency of one's

Certified Professional Coder (CPC) certificate. The individual's commitment to continuous education will guarantee the perpetuation of their skills' relevance and their ability to stay updated with the latest advancements in their respective field.

The present discourse pertains to the subject of remote work opportunities.

The option to engage in remote work or work from other places is a desirable benefit that is highly valued by several individuals employed in the field of medical coding. The aforementioned flexibility has the potential to facilitate the attainment of an improved equilibrium between work and personal life, reduce the duration of commuting, and result in financial savings related to transportation expenses. The likelihood of discovering remote employment opportunities may be enhanced if an individual possesses a Certified Professional Credential (CPC), since some organizations exhibit a hiring bias towards certified professionals when filling such roles.

The Role of Contributions in Enhancing the Delivery of High-Quality Healthcare

In summary, it is imperative to acknowledge that those employed in the domain of medical coding make substantial contributions to the operation of the healthcare system. Accurate coding is essential for several healthcare-related activities, including billing, medical research, obtaining community health information, and healthcare service planning. As a Certified Professional Coder (CPC), your responsibility is in assuring the accuracy and effectiveness of coding operations, so allowing you to actively contribute to the broader healthcare ecosystem.

The journey towards achieving the Certified Professional Coder (CPC) designation takes significant effort and dedication. However, once attaining this milestone, several incentives await individuals. Furthermore, during your tenure in this program, you will have the opportunity to not only acquire information and establish a reputable standing within your area, but also to have a significant impact on the field of healthcare. The journey towards becoming a Certified Professional Coder (CPC) will be characterized by continuous learning and professional growth, leading to a prosperous and fulfilling career trajectory.

The concept of job satisfaction has been a topic of interest and research in the field of organizational psychology. It refers to an individual's subjective evaluation of their overall experience and feelings towards their work. Job satisfaction is influenced

A profession in medical coding may be well-suited for persons who excel in meticulousness and possess problem-solving skills, since it requires a keen focus on detail and the ability to tackle complex issues. The process of determining the suitable codes for each medical intervention and diagnostic has resemblance to the everyday engagement in puzzle-solving activities. Recognizing that one's work has a direct role in enhancing the effectiveness of healthcare services and delivering exceptional patient care may engender a sense of purpose within the profession, therefore constituting an additional advantage.

A wide range of job locations with varying characteristics

Individuals who have obtained their CPC certification are not limited to employment only inside hospital or clinic settings. Proficiency in medical coding is a prerequisite for a wide range of organizations, encompassing insurance corporations, consultancy firms, public health entities, and even law firms specializing in medical affairs. The presence of diversity within the workplace can contribute to the maintenance of job engagement and provide individuals with the chance to discern a working environment that aligns well with their preferences and abilities.

Prospects for an International Career

The CPC certification is grounded on the coding systems employed inside the United States. Nevertheless, the competencies and expertise acquired through the attainment of this certification may be applied to other international code systems. This might potentially create opportunities for work in foreign nations or with multinational healthcare organizations.

The potential for broadening one's professional network

One additional advantage of possessing the CPC certification is the opportunity to join a professional organization like the AAPC (American Academy of Professional Coders). These organizations provide members opportunities to establish new professional relationships, access to educational resources for increasing their knowledge, and support in progressing their careers. Within these professional networks, individuals have the opportunity to establish relationships with other professionals, engage in the sharing of valuable information, and even access mentorship resources to support their career development.

The Role of the Gateway to Management Positions within an Organization

Obtaining a CPC certification might function as a pivotal milestone for persons aspiring to progress their professional trajectories towards managerial positions. Advancement within the coding sector can be achieved by the accumulation of higher levels of education and more professional experience, ultimately leading to managerial positions such as coding manager, health information manager, or head of a coding department. These positions entail a broader scope of responsibilities, a higher remuneration, and the potential to significantly influence the provision of healthcare.

A Lifelong Career

The vocation of coding medical data is expected to be in high demand throughout an individual's professional career. The perpetual need for healthcare experts ensures the continued necessity of medical coders. Furthermore, due to the intricate nature of the healthcare industry and its continuous evolution, the significance of coders' role is poised to further escalate.

In summary, obtaining the CPC certification can serve as an initial milestone towards embarking on a stable and fulfilling career path that has several opportunities for both personal and professional growth. This profession offers not only individual benefits but also the chance to make significant contributions to the area of medicine as a whole.

The American Academy of Professional Coders (AAPC) is widely recognized as a very prominent entity within the domains of medical coding, billing, and healthcare business administration. The institution is widely recognized for its rigorous certification programs, including the renowned Certified Professional Coder (CPC) program.

In relation to the American Academy of Professional Coders (AAPC):

Since its establishment in 1988, the American Academy of Professional Coders (AAPC) has amassed a membership over 200,000 professionals (as per the numbers provided during my most recent training session in September 2021). The primary objective of the company is to further the education of healthcare professionals involved in medical coding, auditing, compliance, and revenue management by providing them with the chance to obtain professional certification.

The American Academy of Professional Coders (AAPC) offers a range of certification programs designed specifically for individuals in various roles within the healthcare industry, including professional coders, medical auditors, compliance officers, and practice managers. These programs aim to enhance the existing standards of healthcare business operations by ensuring the attainment of high levels of competence, ethical conduct, and professional proficiency.

The membership in the American Academy of Professional Coders (AAPC) offers several benefits and advantages to those seeking to further their professional development in the field of medical coding and billing.

There exist several benefits associated with membership in the American Academy of Professional Coders (AAPC), which can be summarized as follows:

1. One of the key advantages is the ability to establish professional contacts. By joining the American Academy of Professional Coders (AAPC), individuals get the opportunity to connect with a diverse network of healthcare business professionals hailing from various regions within the United States and internationally. The aforementioned network has promising potential as a valuable resource for accessing professional support, facilitating the sharing of information, and exploring opportunities for career progression.

2. The AAPC offers a wide range of continuing education programs to its members, including as webinars, on-demand events, and local chapter meetings, in order to support ongoing training and education. These types of activities are sometimes included while calculating Continuing Education Units (CEUs), which are necessary for maintaining the validity of one's certification.

3. The AAPC offers its members opportunities for career advancement, job search support, and professional development. These tools may provide significant assistance to individuals at any point in their professional growth, regardless of whether they are in the early stages of their career or striving for advancement.

4. Members of the AAPC are entitled to substantial discounts on certification tests and related products, such as study guides, practice exams, and the Medical Coding Training CPC program provided by the AAPC. These discounted prices allow members the opportunity to access these resources at a reduced cost.

5. [Recent Developments and Industry News]: As a member, you will receive regular updates on the most recent industry trends, modifications in coding standards, and other relevant news that aligns with your interests. This resource has the potential to assist individuals in staying abreast of the most recent advancements within their respective fields of expertise.

The availability of the Code Lookup Tool offered by the American Academy of Professional Coders (AAPC). This tool is a comprehensive online resource that may be utilized to search for CPT, HCPCS, ICD-10-CM, and ICD-9-CM codes. The utilization of this tool has the potential to enhance one's performance in their professional responsibilities and facilitate their readiness for certification examinations.

Being a member of the AAPC might offer several advantages for one's professional trajectory. The healthcare business sector offers a range of tools, support, and opportunities that have the potential to facilitate success in this industry.

The process of becoming a member of the AAPC is rather straightforward. The below enumeration outlines the sequential procedures that must be adhered to:

1. Access the Official Website of the AAPC: The initial step is navigating to the official website of the American Academy of Professional Coders (AAPC).

2. Select the Membership Category That Best Fits Your Needs The AAPC offers many membership types. Working professionals have the opportunity to join in an individual membership, while students who are currently enrolled in an educational program can choose for a student membership. Prior to making a decision, it is advisable to thoroughly evaluate the advantages provided by each alternative.

3. Please include the requested information in the Application Form. Once the appropriate membership option has been determined, the subsequent step involves completing the application process on the website. Upon commencing the completion of this form, you will be required to provide your personal information, educational history, and professional background.

4. Proceed with the payment for the membership fee. Upon completion of the application form, it is mandatory for you to remit the membership fee. The cost of membership exhibits significant variation contingent upon the specific type of membership chosen. Based on the available data as of September 2021, it was observed that the annual fee for an individual membership amounted to $175, whilst a student membership incurred an annual fee of $90.

5. Review and Submit: Carefully examine the information you have submitted and thereafter submit your application. Once the membership application and payment have undergone processing, a confirmation email will be dispatched to you, with detailed information pertaining to your membership.

It is essential to bear in mind that mere membership does not inherently provide the status of a certified professional. In order to obtain the CPC designation, it is important to achieve a satisfactory score on the Certified Professional Coder (CPC) test. In order to facilitate your test preparation, the AAPC provides a range of educational resources and study aids to support your exam readiness.

It is advisable to consistently verify the most up-to-date information on the official website of the American Academy of Professional Coders (AAPC) in order to ascertain the utmost accuracy of the facts. It is important to note that the cost and methodology may have undergone major changes subsequent to my knowledge cutoff in 2021.

How to Use This Study Guide Effectively

The process of acquiring knowledge may be likened as embarking upon a vast expanse of information, akin to the act of setting sail on an ocean. Commencing a learning endeavor bears resemblance to this analogy. An efficient study guide serves as a navigational tool, aiding individuals in traversing complex subject matter and facilitating their successful attainment of desired learning outcomes. However, what specific methods may be employed to optimize the efficiency of this tool? Optimal utilization of the study guide can be attained by adhering to the following recommendations.

It is vital to ensure a thorough understanding of one's study guide.

Prior to immersing oneself in the subject matter, it is advisable to allocate a certain amount of time to familiarize oneself with the structure and arrangement of the study guide. The user is advised to thoroughly analyze the table of contents, synopses of individual chapters, and any introductory or descriptive statements that may be present. This document will furnish you with a comprehensive overview of the content that is included, along with a detailed elucidation of its organizational structure.

Develop a structured timetable for your academic pursuits and adhere to it diligently.

Once a comprehensive comprehension of the issues covered in the handbook has been acquired, it is advisable to establish a study regimen. The guide should be divided into manageable sections, with a designated amount of time allocated for each segment. It is vital to ensure that one's plan include many instances of review in order to consolidate the acquired information.

Active reading is a form of reading that requires engagement and participation from the reader.

Engaging in active reading entails more than simply glancing over the textual content with one's eyes. Demonstrate a proactive engagement with the subject matter. The user is advised to identify and highlight the portions that are most applicable to their needs. They are encouraged to make annotations in the margins and provide a summary of each section using their own words. The retention of knowledge is enhanced as a result of the active engagement exhibited by the participants.

Utilize all supplementary components.

Most study aids are often accompanied by additional resources such as quizzes, flashcards, and practice questions. Harness their maximum capabilities. Internships provide individuals the chance to apply acquired knowledge and skills, therefore providing a tangible measure of personal growth and progress.

In conjunction with the accessibility of alternative resources

Although the provided study guide is indeed a comprehensive resource, it is not advisable to depend only on it. Utilize the aforementioned resources, including the prescribed coursework, textbooks, and online materials, in conjunction with one another. This will provide a more profound and extensive understanding of the topic matter.

It is recommended to engage in regular review of the subject matter.

Regularly reviewing material is crucial for the retention of information in memory. Consistently engaging in the practice of reviewing one's notes and extracting the main points from each section might enhance the retention of information. The process of repetition facilitates the transfer of knowledge from short-term memory to long-term memory.

It is important to prioritize the incorporation of regular breaks into one's routine.

It is important to allocate sufficient time for the brain to unwind and assimilate the information it has received. During the period of academic engagement, it is important to allocate regular intervals for taking breaks. The Pomodoro Technique is a time management approach that advocates for allocating 25 minutes to focused study followed by a 5-minute interval of rest. This particular tactic has significant popularity.

Maintaining Optimal Health

The status of one's physical health has an impact on their ability to learn effectively. It is essential to ensure that an adequate quantity of sleep is obtained, a nutritious diet is maintained, and consistent physical exercise is included into one's daily routine.

It is important to note that the primary goal is not only to finish the book, but rather to thoroughly understand and assimilate the content. Engaging in this practice will not only enhance your academic achievements, but it will also foster personal growth, expanding your knowledge and cultivating a comprehensive understanding.

One of the most appealing attributes of a study guide is its capacity for adaptation. Individuals have the freedom to modify and apply this resource according to their own learning style, specific requirements, and personal schedule. While certain individuals may find it advantageous to engage in a comprehensive review of the guide initially to get a holistic understanding, others may find it more advantageous to conduct a meticulous examination of each topic before on to the subsequent one. There is no universally applicable approach that can be employed in all situations. The key to success is in maintaining active engagement, ensuring consistency, and tailoring the approach to one's individual preferences. The study guide transcends its utilitarian purpose and becomes a multifaceted role. It serves as a dependable companion on one's journey towards acquiring knowledge.

The utilization of flashcards, a versatile and efficient educational aid, can facilitate the consolidation of acquired knowledge and enhance memory retrieval. Here are few strategies that can effectively facilitate the integration of these methods into one's regular study regimen:

1. A Concise Overview of Recent Developments:
Incorporating the practice of reviewing flashcards into one's daily study regimen is recommended. Regular exposure to the information facilitates the transfer of knowledge from one's working memory to their long-term memory.

2. The Concept of Spaced Repetition Intervals:
The approach to learning involves reviewing previously acquired knowledge with progressively larger intervals as time elapses. To begin the learning process, allocate a portion of the study session to repetitively reviewing a newly created flashcard. Subsequently, it is advisable to do a thorough review on the subsequent day, followed by subsequent reviews on the second and fourth days, and so on. Research has shown that the utilization of this particular method leads to enhanced long-term memory preservation of information.

3. Recall exercise is as follows:
Prior to flipping the flashcard, it is advisable to engage in a cognitive process of recalling and retrieving the information from one's memory, rather than only relying on reading the content. Active engagement with material leads to enhanced memory retention.

4. One way to provide variability in a card game is by shuffling the deck thoroughly.
The act of shuffling flashcards can help mitigate the building of cognitive associations between material and its sequential presentation order in the brain. This finding substantiates the notion that you are retrieving information alone, without any external aid.

5. Conduct a comprehensive analysis and deconstruction of intricate concepts: When confronted with complex concepts, it might be advantageous to deconstruct those concepts into their constituent pieces and organize them into a collection of flashcards. As a result of this, the topic may potentially be rendered more comprehensible and facilitate improved retention.

6. One effective strategy is to incorporate visual aids into the presentation. Incorporate visual aids such as images, graphs, or sections with color coding into your flashcards. The utilization of visual aids can facilitate the enhanced retention of knowledge.

Collaborative research refers to the process of conducting scientific investigations or studies in which several individuals or groups work together towards a common research goal. This approach involves pooling resources,

When engaging in a collaborative study session, it is advisable to consider the utilization of flashcards. One potential approach to enhance the studying session's dynamism and entertainment value for both individuals involved is to engage in reciprocal testing.

Carry Them With You: An Exploration of the Eighth Element

Carrying flashcards at all times allows individuals to utilize normally unproductive periods, such as waiting in queues or taking work breaks, to engage in a rapid review of the subject matter.

One effective strategy to enhance learning is the utilization of digital flashcards.

Numerous websites and mobile applications may be found on the internet, offering users the ability to create digital flashcards. There are several advantages associated with these tools, such as the inclusion of pre-existing algorithms for spaced repetition, convenient portability, and the ability to integrate multimedia elements.

By using these strategies, not only will the efficiency of your study sessions be enhanced, but also the effectiveness of your flashcards will be heightened. It is crucial to bear in mind that the primary goal is not only to finish all of the cards, but rather to absorb and remember the information. In the realm of education, the superiority of quality over quantity is consistently evident.

Book 1: Medical Terminology

Common Medical Terms by Body System

A comprehensive understanding of the several medical terminologies employed in contemporary healthcare is a fundamental need for any occupation within the healthcare sector. Possessing this information will facilitate effective communication among colleagues, enhance comprehension of patient data, and enable the delivery of improved patient care. This chapter will undertake an examination of many widely used medical terms, organized according to the respective bodily systems.

The cardiovascular system, consisting of the heart and blood vessels, plays a crucial role in the circulation of blood throughout the body.

The cardiovascular system, consisting of the heart and blood vessels, is responsible for the vital task of pumping and circulating blood throughout the whole body.

Arrhythmia is the term used to describe an anomaly or disruption in the regular cardiac rhythm.
Atherosclerosis refers to the pathological process characterized by the deposition of lipids and cholesterol inside the luminal surface of arterial walls, ultimately resulting in arterial stenosis and potential occlusion.
Myocardial infarction, commonly referred to as a heart attack, occurs as a result of diminished blood flow to a specific region of the heart.

The respiratory system facilitates the process of gas exchange, allowing people to inhale oxygen and exhale carbon dioxide.

Bronchial tube inflammation, known as bronchitis, occurs in the airways responsible for facilitating the movement of air to and from the lungs. The medical term used to describe this disease is bronchitis.
Pneumonia is a pathological condition characterized by the inflammation of the pulmonary alveoli, affecting either unilateral or bilateral lung involvement.
Tachypnea is a clinical manifestation defined by an increased respiratory rate, commonly observed in adults when the breathing frequency exceeds 20 breaths per minute.

The gastrointestinal system, often known as the digestive system, refers to the collection of organs and processes involved in the digestion and absorption of

The aforementioned system is responsible for the process of food digestion, the uptake of essential nutrients, and the excretion of waste materials.

Cholecystitis refers to the inflammatory condition affecting the gallbladder, primarily attributed to the presence of gallstones.
Intestinal and gastric inflammation, typically attributed to viral or bacterial infections, is a prevailing condition. The medical term for this ailment is gastroenteritis.
Hepatitis is an inflammatory condition affecting the liver, primarily caused by viral infections.

The nervous system is a complex network of cells and tissues that facilitates communication and coordination inside the body.

The neurological system use electrical impulses to regulate bodily functions. The human nervous system consists of two main components: the central nervous system (CNS) and the peripheral nervous system (PNS). The CNS is formed of the brain and spinal cord, while the PNS is comprised of the nerves that are situated outside of the CNS.

Neuropathy is the medical term used to describe the state of having impaired or malfunctioning nerves. Epilepsy is a neurological disorder that is defined by the occurrence of recurrent episodes of seizure activity.
Parkinson's disease is a neurodegenerative disorder characterized by progressive motor deficits.

The aforementioned system provides the human body with its structural form, while also offering essential functions such as support, stability, and the ability to engage in movement.

Arthritis refers to the inflammatory condition affecting one or more joints, resulting in pain and stiffness within the afflicted joint(s).
Osteoporosis is a pathological condition characterized by the progressive loss of bone mass and density, resulting in increased fragility and decreased structural integrity of the skeletal system.
Tendinitis refers to the inflammatory or irritative condition of a tendon, typically resulting from repetitive, low-intensity impact on the afflicted area.

The topic of discussion pertains to the system of endocrine glands.

The endocrine system comprises a collection of glands that synthesize and secrete hormones to regulate many physiological processes inside the body, such as metabolism, growth, and sexual function.

Diabetes is a persistent medical disorder characterized by insufficient production of insulin or impaired use of available insulin inside the body.
The user's text does not provide any information to be rewritten in an academic manner. The medical terminology used to describe the disorder characterized by the overproduction of thyroid hormone by the thyroid gland.
The user's text does not contain any information to rewrite. Addison's disease is a medical illness characterized by insufficient hormone production in the adrenal glands.

Gaining proficiency in medical terminology can be likened to the process of studying a foreign language. Initially, one would see it as an arduous task; but, through diligent study and regular application, one will ascertain that these principles assimilate effortlessly within a short span of time. Applying these principles within a given situation consistently is an effective approach for acquiring and retaining knowledge. It is advisable to actively incorporate these new vocabulary words into your everyday language, document them in phrases, or employ flashcards as a means of regularly reviewing and reinforcing your knowledge of them.

It is noteworthy that a substantial portion of medical terminology has its origins in Latin and Greek languages. An illustration may be seen in the term "myocardial," whereby the prefix "myo-" denotes muscle and the suffix "cardiac" pertains to the heart. Consequently, acquiring knowledge of prevalent Latin and Greek roots, prefixes, and suffixes might facilitate the comprehension of medical terminology. By employing this approach, it is possible to infer the meaning of an unfamiliar word by utilizing contextual clues that are readily accessible.

The integumentary system encompasses the skin, hair, nails, and associated glands responsible for producing sweat and oil. The aforementioned system plays a crucial role in facilitating the body's defense mechanisms against external dangers and regulating its internal temperature.

Dermatitis refers to an inflammatory condition affecting the integumentary system, characterized by pruritus, erythema, and the formation of cutaneous ulcers.
Melanoma is a malignant kind of cutaneous neoplasm originating from melanocytes, the cells responsible for synthesizing melanin. These cells represent the initial stage of the illness.
Psoriasis is a chronic dermatological disorder characterized by dysregulated immune response, resulting in accelerated epidermal cell turnover and the manifestation of scaly plaques and erythematous patches on the skin.

The urinary bladder is an integral component of the human urinary system.

The urinary system is comprised of several components, namely the kidneys, ureters, bladder, and urethra. The aforementioned system is accountable for the process of blood filtration and the elimination of waste substances from the human body, which are afterwards expelled in the form of urine.

Cystitis refers to the inflammatory condition of the bladder, typically caused by an infection inside the urinary system.
Renal failure is a pathological state characterized by the kidneys' inability to effectively carry out their physiological role of eliminating metabolic waste substances from the bloodstream.
The user's text does not provide any information to rewrite in an academic manner. Urolithiasis is a medical disorder characterized by the development of calculi, commonly referred to as stones, inside the renal system, including the kidneys, bladder, or urethra.

The immune system plays a crucial role in safeguarding the body from pathogenic microorganisms that have the potential to induce illness.

Autoimmune illness is characterized by the immune system's misidentification of the body's own cells as foreign entities, leading to an erroneous attack against these cells. This phenomenon has the potential to result in a range of significant health consequences.
The term "immunodeficiency" pertains to a medical state characterized by a significant reduction or complete absence of the body's innate ability to defend against infectious diseases.
Lymphoma is a group of hematological malignancies that arise from lymphocytes, a specific kind of leukocyte.

Furthermore, it is important to acknowledge the significance of the reproductive system, as it assumes the responsibility of facilitating the production of subsequent generations within the species.

Endometriosis is a medically distressing condition characterized by the ectopic growth of endometrial-like tissue, resembling the endometrium lining of the uterus, outside the confines of the uterine cavity. Prostatitis is a common condition characterized by the enlargement and inflammation of the prostate gland, leading to frequent discomfort or difficulty while urination. This medical ailment is often known as prostatitis.
Infertility is characterized as the inability to achieve pregnancy after engaging in consistent sexual activity for a duration of one year or longer, without employing any kind of contraception.

These terminologies constitute a little fraction of the comprehensive vocabulary employed within the medical field. To enhance your comprehension of medical information and effectively convey it, it is advantageous to acquaint yourself with these and other often used terms. It is important to bear in mind that although the act of memorizing words can be advantageous, the paramount aspect is to possess a comprehensive understanding of the significance of each term, as well as its applicability in various situations. The following factors will ultimately contribute to one's success in the healthcare profession. When engaging in the process of acquiring new knowledge, it might prove advantageous to refer to educational resources such as medical dictionaries, textbooks, and reputable online platforms. When encountering an unfamiliar term, it is advisable to seek further information in order to enhance one's understanding.

This analysis will examine commonly used medical terminology related to the sensory system, encompassing the eyes, ears, and lymphatic system.

The concept of the "System of Sensation" refers to the complex network of physiological processes and neural pathways involved in the perception and interpretation of sensory information by the human body

The sensory system comprises visual perception, auditory perception, gustatory perception, olfactory perception, and tactile perception. In this part, our focus will be on terminology that is relevant to both visual and auditory perception.

Astigmatism refers to a condition characterized by an irregularity in the curvature of the cornea or lens of the eye, resulting in visual distortion or blurriness.
The term "glaucoma" encompasses a group of ocular disorders that have the potential to induce harm to the optic nerve. The primary cause of this injury is commonly attributed to abnormally elevated intraocular pressure.
Tinnitus is a prevalent condition often described as a perception of sound in the ears, commonly characterized as a ringing sensation. Nevertheless, it can also manifest as other auditory sensations such as roaring, clicking, hissing, or buzzing. The user's text does not provide any information to rewrite in an academic manner. Tinnitus is a prevalent ailment frequently characterized by the perception of a ringing sensation in the auditory system.
The user's text does not provide any information to be rewritten in an academic manner. Otitis Media is a medical term used to describe the inflammatory or infectious condition affecting the middle ear, which is recognized as the primary etiology of ear discomfort.

The lymphatic system

The lymphatic system constitutes an integral part of the immune system. The lymphatic system comprises a complex network of lymphatic vessels that facilitate the transportation of lymph, a transparent bodily fluid, towards the cardiac region.

Lymphedema is a persistent condition defined by edema in the body's tissues, resulting from either lymphatic system damage or obstruction. Lymphadenopathy is a medical disorder characterized by abnormal size or consistency of the lymph nodes.
Lymphoma is a kind of cancer that affects the lymphatic system. As previously mentioned, lymphoma is a malignancy that initially arises in cells belonging to the body's immune system.

In conclusion, it is vital to examine some frequently employed terms across various body systems.

According to medical terminology, a condition is classified as acute when it manifests abruptly, exhibits a considerable degree of severity, yet has a relatively short duration.
The term "chronic" refers to a medical condition or illness that exhibits enduring repercussions over an extended duration, also referred to as "persistent."
Idiopathic diseases or disorders are characterized by an unknown or incompletely understood underlying cause.
A prognosis refers to a prediction or projection regarding the expected progression and ultimate result of a medical condition.
The term "benign" refers to a condition or characteristic that is neither harmful or threatening in nature. The term "benign" is employed to characterize situations where there is no adverse impact. For example, a tumor that lacks malignancy is referred to be benign.
The term "malignant" is employed to characterize pathological conditions characterized by the uncontrolled division of abnormal cells and their ability to invade neighboring tissues. Moreover, malignant cells has the capacity to disseminate throughout the organism by means of the circulatory and lymphatic systems.

The comprehension of medical terminology can provide challenges, despite its inherent rationality and systematic nature. Once an individual possesses a comprehensive understanding of the core constituents of a word, namely its roots, prefixes, and suffixes, they will be equipped to employ this knowledge in order to comprehend a wide range of phrases. Devoting oneself to the study of medical language is a highly valuable pursuit that merits considerable investment of time and effort. Engaging in healthcare education and pursuing a career in the healthcare business not only offers benefits in terms of academic growth and professional prospects, but also presents the chance to enhance one's understanding as a patient or caregiver.

Word Parts (Prefixes, Suffixes, and Combining Forms)

Upon embarking on an exploration of medical terminology, it becomes evident in a very short span of time that several terms are akin to intricate puzzles, formed by the amalgamation of diverse word parts including prefixes, suffixes, and combining forms. By comprehending these constituent elements, a seemingly intricate and daunting concept may be turned into a comprehensible and meaningful entity.

The topic of discussion pertains to the recognition of prefixes, specifically focusing on the comprehension of prefixes.

The insertion of a prefix, a word component placed at the beginning of a word, has the potential to modify the meaning of the term. In the realm of medical terminology, the subsequent are a few prefixes that are frequently employed:

The prefix "hyper-" denotes a state or condition that is situated beyond or beyond a certain threshold, as well as an excessive quantity or degree. An illustrative instance pertains to the medical phenomenon recognized as hyperglycemia, denoting an anomalous elevation in glucose levels in the bloodstream.
The prefix hypo- denotes a state of being "under," "below," or "deficient." The prefix hyper- has an antonym. The word "hypotension" refers to a condition characterized by a blood pressure that is notably lower than the average range. The user's text is already academic. The prefix "dys-" is employed to denote challenges, distress, or an anomalous operation. An illustration of this phenomenon is the medical ailment referred to as "dysphagia," which encompasses challenges in the act of swallowing.

An Exposition on the Interpretation of Suffixes

The addition of a suffix to the end of a word might result in a modification of its meaning. The subsequent instances illustrate commonly employed suffixes:

The presence of inflammation is denoted by the suffix "-itis," which is derived from the Greek word "itis." As an illustration, the medical term "arthritis" denotes the pathological state characterized by inflammation of the joints.
The term "oma" is commonly utilized in medical terminology to refer to a tumor or other form of neoplasm. To provide an example, a carcinoma refers to a type of neoplastic growth characterized by its cancerous or malignant nature.
The suffix "-ectomy" is utilized to denote the necessity of surgical excision, which refers to the process of surgically removing a certain anatomical structure or tissue. An illustration of this phenomenon may be observed in the medical treatment commonly referred to as a "appendectomy," which entails the surgical extraction of the appendix.

22

The process of integrating many forms into coherent navigational pathways.

An instance of a combining form is observed when a word root is appended with a vowel at its end, or when a vowel is affixed to the beginning of a word root or suffix. The vowel 'o' is utilized more frequently than any other vowel in combining forms. Several examples are as follows:

Cardiovascular: Pertaining to or pertaining to the heart. When combined with additional morphemes, it gives rise to lexical units such as "cardiology," which pertains to the scientific investigation of cardiac ailments, and "cardiomegaly," which denotes the pathological condition characterized by an abnormal increase in the size of the heart.

The user's text does not provide any information to rewrite in an academic manner. The prefix "hemato" denotes a relationship or association with blood. The combining form in question may be observed in terms such as "hematoma," denoting the collection of blood within tissue that subsequently coagulates to form a firm swelling, and "hematology," which pertains to the examination of the characteristics, functioning, and abnormalities of the blood.

When attempting to decode unfamiliar medical vocabulary, it is advantageous to possess comprehension of the semantic components comprising these expressions. The process of deconstructing words into their individual components often allows for the inference of the overall meaning of the term. Consider, for instance, the term "hypoglycemia" as an exemplification. The term "hypoglycemia" may be deconstructed by analyzing its constituent parts, including the prefix "hypo-," denoting "below" or "under," the prefix "glyc/o," signifying "sugar," and the suffix "-emia," indicating a condition that impacts the blood.

The process of obtaining medical terminology using this approach can be likened to the process of acquiring the foundational grammar of a new language. Acquiring a foundational understanding of verbs, nouns, and adjectives can facilitate the construction of sentences in a novel linguistic system. Similarly, acquiring knowledge of fundamental prefixes, suffixes, and combining forms can facilitate the understanding and proficiency in medical terminology.

It is crucial to bear in mind that the practice of medical language acquisition is of utmost significance. Regularly examining these word components and making a conscious effort to identify them inside medical words is of utmost importance. The more one's familiarity with these components, the easier it becomes to grasp and retain medical terminology.

It is important to note that while the majority of medical terms adhere to this pattern, there exist certain exceptions. Certain words may not be easily broken down into the standard prefixes, roots, and suffixes, whilst other words may possess meanings that have undergone changes through time or do not strictly conform to established linguistic standards. To effectively retain this information, it is necessary to engage in repeated exposure.

In conclusion, it is advisable to develop a routine of verifying one's understanding of medical language prior to use it in any context, with a special emphasis on healthcare-related situations. Misinterpretation of medical terminology can lead to errors in the administration of patient care. Given the aforementioned circumstances, it is advisable to seek guidance from authoritative medical dictionaries or subject matter specialists if one encounters ambiguity regarding the interpretation of a medical term.

In order to have a deeper understanding of medical terminology, it is necessary to explore supplementary prefixes, suffixes, and combining forms and analyze their use within the field.

The incorporation of additional prefixes

Prior to completing the whole reading of a medical term, a proficient comprehension of its prefixes enables one to have a reasonable concept of its intended reference. Presented here are further illustrations:

The prefix "Brady-" denotes a state or quality of being characterized by slowness or sluggishness. An illustration of this concept may be found in the medical word "bradycardia," which denotes a cardiac rhythm characterized by a heart rate much below the average range.
The prefix tachy-, denoting "rapid," functions as the opposite of the brady- prefix. An illustrative instance involves a medical condition referred to as "tachycardia," which is a circumstance whereby the heart exhibits a substantially elevated rate of beating compared to its typical rhythm.
The aforementioned prefix is employed to indicate a state of being extensive or having considerable dimensions. The term "macro" is most frequently utilized in this context. The medical condition known as "macrocephaly" refers to an atypically enlarged cranium.

The presence of a larger quantity of suffixes

The classification of a technique, sickness, issue, or disease may often be ascertained based on its suffix. Furthermore, the use of supplementary visual aids encompasses the subsequent examples:

The suffix "-osis" is commonly used to indicate the presence of a certain condition, often associated with a pathological state, such as a disease. An illustration of this may be seen in the condition referred to as scoliosis, which is distinguished by atypical curvature of the vertebral column.

The user's text does not contain any information. The suffix "-graphy" serves as an indicator of a technique employed for the purpose of documenting or recording. The suffix "-graphy" is commonly used in academic discourse to denote a field of study or a method of recording or representing information Electrocardiography, often known as ECG, is a diagnostic technique used to capture and analyze the electrical impulses generated by the heart. The name "electrocardiography" specifically denotes the process of capturing these electrical signals.

The user's text does not contain any information to rewrite. The suffix "-pathy" is utilized to denote a medical condition or ailment in its semantic sense. One such ailment is commonly known as "neuropathy," which encompasses both illnesses and disorders that impact the peripheral nerves.

Additional Combinations of Forms

The discipline of medical language commonly use combining words to denote qualities, conditions, or specific bodily systems. Presented here are further illustrations:

The prefix "cephalo" denotes a relationship or association with the anatomical region known as the head. As an illustration, the term "cephalalgia" is a medical ailment characterized by a sensation of pain in the head, often known as a headache. Similarly, "hydrocephalus" is a medical condition characterized by the abnormal buildup of cerebrospinal fluid inside the brain, resulting in the enlargement of the head.

The user's text does not provide any information to rewrite in an academic manner. The term "osteo" is used to indicate a connection or association with the skeletal system. The combining form in question may be observed in phrases such as "osteoporosis," denoting a condition characterized by the fragility and weakness of bones, and "osteopathy," referring to a kind of alternative medicine that emphasizes the physical manipulation of muscle tissue and bones.

A comprehensive understanding of medical language may be achieved by acquiring knowledge of word components and their common usage. As an illustration, the term "osteoporosis" may be deconstructed into its constituent parts, namely "oste/o," denoting bone, and "-porosis," signifying porous, so yielding the expression "porous bones." The following is a concise portrayal of the given condition.

Acquiring proficiency in medical terminology entails more than just rote memorization; instead, it necessitates a comprehensive understanding of the underlying principles that inform the language of medicine. By dedicating additional time to familiarizing oneself with these linguistic components, individuals will find it far easier to grasp the terminology employed by healthcare professionals.

However, it is crucial to acknowledge that medical terminology serves as a valuable instrument for promoting effective communication within healthcare environments. It is often advisable to pursue clarification when encountering a term that is not completely comprehended, as opposed to potentially encountering misunderstandings or misinterpretations. In the medical domain, the consequences are significant, and effective communication characterized by clarity and precision can have life-or-death implications.

In conclusion, it is essential to acknowledge that language undergoes evolution through time, and medical terminology is not exempt from this phenomenon. As the area of medical research progresses, novel terminology is consistently being introduced. Healthcare professionals have an ongoing need to stay updated on the latest modifications and additions to medical terminology. A comprehensive comprehension of fundamental components, such as prefixes, suffixes, and combining forms, can greatly enhance your ability to comprehend and assimilate unfamiliar medical terminology.

Further examples of how forms might be included in medical terminology. It is crucial to bear in mind that the composition of combining forms often involves a root word and a vowel, with the letter 'o' being the most commonly used. These forms serve the purpose of connecting multiple roots or a root and a suffix.

1. The combining form "neur/o" is commonly used to refer to the phrase "nerve" or "nervous system." An illustrative instance is the designation "neurologist," denoting a medical practitioner with specialized expertise in addressing conditions that impact the neurological system.

2. The combining forms "pneum" and "pneumon" pertain to the presence of air, the lungs, or the respiratory system. An instance of a sickness known as "pneumonia" results in the inflammation of the air sacs located in either one or both lungs. This inflammatory response might manifest in either of the lungs.

3. The prefix hepato is used to denote the liver in this sentence. The term "hepatitis," denoting the inflammatory condition of the liver, serves as an illustrative instance of a lexeme employing this particular morphological element.

4. The combining form "cardi/o" is commonly utilized in reference to the circulatory system, specifically pertaining to the heart. An illustration of this phenomenon may be observed in the medical domain, specifically in the context of a pathological disease referred to as "cardiomyopathy." This term encompasses a range of illnesses that exert an impact on the myocardium, the muscular tissue of the heart.

5. The term "arthr" is used to denote the anatomical structures known as joints inside the human body. Consider, for example, the medical condition referred to

as "arthritis," which is distinguished by the presence of inflammation in one or many joints.

6. The combining form "gastr/o" is used to denote the anatomical organ commonly known as the stomach. An illustration of this phenomenon may be observed in the medical disease commonly referred to as "gastritis," denoting the inflammatory state of the gastric mucosa.

The terms "Dermato" and "Dermo" are both related to the subject matter of the integumentary system. To illustrate, the term "dermatitis" denotes an inflammatory condition affecting the integumentary system.

The combining form ophthalm/o pertains to entities or concepts that are related to the anatomical structure and functions of the human eye. An illustrative instance is the "ophthalmoscope," a device that enables the examination of the inside anatomical structures of the eye.

The names "hemato" or "hemo" are used to denote blood in their respective linguistic forms. An illustration of a medical specialty referred to as "hematology" entails a concentrated examination of blood, alongside the organs responsible for blood production and the ailments that impact blood.

The combining form used to denote the kidney is nephro. A nephrologist is an exemplar of a healthcare practitioner who specializes in the diagnosis and treatment of kidney disorders.

It is vital to bear in mind that acquiring knowledge of these combining forms can provide a solid foundation for the interpretation of medical terminology. By acquiring these essential components, individuals will be able to assemble the meanings of complex medical terminology, hence enhancing their ability to understand and communicate effectively within a healthcare setting.

Medical Abbreviations

In the realm of health and medicine, timeliness and efficacy can significantly impact outcomes. As a consequence, specialists in the medical field possess a necessity for medical abbreviations, which serve as a type of concise notation enabling them to record intricate concepts in a more expedient method. Nevertheless, those lacking familiarity with this abbreviation may see it as a whole distinct linguistic system. Let us delve into the intricacies of medical abbreviations in order to enhance your expertise in these concise linguistic tools.

Abbreviations utilized within the medical domain encompass a concise form of linguistic expressions or terminologies, denoted by a condensed amalgamation of symbols and letters. Medical environments, ranging from clinics and hospitals to research centers, demonstrate extensive utilization of these technologies. Having a comprehensive understanding of these acronyms is crucial for anyone employed in the healthcare sector, particularly those working as medical coders and billers.

In order to comprehend medical abbreviations, it is important to acknowledge that they serve as substitutes for a diverse range of medical terminology. Let us examine some other types, shall we?

The subject of discussion pertains to anatomical terminology. These acronyms pertain to distinct anatomical regions of the human organism. As an illustration, the abbreviation "ABD" is commonly employed to denote the anatomical word "abdomen," whereas "AC" is frequently utilized as an abbreviation for "acromioclavicular," which refers to a specific joint located in the shoulder region.

- Diagnostic and Procedural Terminology: These acronyms are often employed as abbreviations for medical procedures or diagnostic terms. As an illustration, the acronym "CABG" denotes a particular cardiac surgical procedure recognized as coronary artery bypass graft, whereas "CAD" designates a medical condition identified as coronary artery disease.

The terminologies employed to represent various units of measurement in medical testing are commonly known as "Measurement Units." For example, the abbreviations "mg" and "L" represent the units of milligrams and liters, correspondingly.

- Anatomical Terminology for Directions and Locations: The following acronyms are utilized to denote anatomical directions and particular locations on the human body. As an illustrative example, the abbreviation "PO" is an acronym for the Latin term "per os," which translates to "by mouth," whereas "IV" is an abbreviation for "intravenous."

- Vocabulary Pertaining to Frequency and Duration: These acronyms are employed to indicate the frequency and duration of a therapy. As an illustration, the abbreviation 'q4h' is an abbreviated form of the phrase 'every four hours,' but 'prn' is an abbreviated form of the Latin term 'pro re nata,' which translates to 'as needed.'

Upon acquiring knowledge about the various types of phrases that are subject to abbreviation, it is imperative to consider the following essential considerations while dealing with abbreviations in the medical domain:

The semantic interpretation of an abbreviation might vary contingent upon the contextual environment in which it is employed. The consideration of context is of paramount significance. The acronym 'CAP' can have several meanings depending on the context. It may refer to Community-Acquired Pneumonia or to the College of American Pathologists.

Standardization efforts have been undertaken by several healthcare institutions to mitigate the potential for patients to receive inaccurate information. These initiatives involve the establishment of standardized compendiums including approved acronyms. If there is any ambiguity regarding an abbreviation, it is advisable to consult one of the available lists.

The utilization of certain acronyms carries a potential for misunderstanding, hence leading to errors in the provision of medical treatment. An instance of potential confusion arises between the abbreviations "QD" (signifying "every day") and "QID" (indicating "four times a day"). Consequently, several institutions recommend the unambiguous articulation of instructions as a means to mitigate potential hazards.

To acquire proficiency in medical acronyms, engaging in regular practice is vital. Enhance your familiarity with prevalent abbreviations by engaging in frequent self-quizzing sessions with comprehensive lists of such abbreviations. When reviewing medical data, it is essential to proactively research any abbreviations that are unfamiliar to ensure comprehensive understanding.
Given the prevalence of the digital age, there exists a wide array of online resources and mobile applications that can aid individuals in acquiring proficiency in medical abbreviations. These tools have the potential to enhance the learning experience by introducing interactive elements like as flashcards, quizzes, and games, hence increasing engagement and interest.

Fortunately, it is not necessary to memorize all of these items, even if the endeavor may appear daunting. Instead, it is advisable to prioritize the acquisition of vocabulary that is often employed within the specific domains of profession or education in which you are engaged. The below suggestions might provide assistance in navigating the vast realm of medical acronyms.

Exploring the Enigmas of the Cipher

When faced with an unfamiliar abbreviation, it is conceivable that one may achieve comprehension by deconstructing it into its constituent parts. Consider, for instance, the acronym MI, which represents the medical term "myocardial infarction" in its entirety. Those who possess knowledge of Latin etymology would recognize that the prefix 'myo-' pertains to muscular tissue, the term 'cardial' is associated with the heart, and 'infarction' signifies the necrosis of tissue resulting from inadequate blood supply. Hence, myocardial infarction denotes the occurrence of necrosis in cardiac tissue, often recognized as a myocardial infarction or heart attack.

Stay updated with the latest information.

The utilization of abbreviations in the field of medicine is subject to change and is not considered permanent. A continuous influx of novel terms is being introduced, together with the gradual obsolescence and potential semantic evolution of certain preexisting terms. It is important to remain well-informed about the latest updates, especially in the domain of medical coding, where accuracy has significant significance. It is advisable to consistently engage in active engagement within respected medical forums and regularly consult reliable medical resources.

Repetition and extensive practice are essential in order to enhance proficiency.

Consistent practice is necessary for attaining proficiency in medical acronyms, much to the need of practice in acquiring a new language. Integrate these strategies into your routine work, employ flashcards for the purpose of reviewing, and engage in the practice of reading case notes or medical reports that feature abbreviations. Over time, you will acquire a comprehensive understanding and aptitude in using these acronyms.

Cautionary Notice: Impending Peril

Despite the potential time-saving benefits associated with the utilization of medical acronyms, their incorrect usage may heighten the probability of misinterpretations. The Institute for Safe prescription Practices (ISMP) maintains a list of abbreviations, acronyms, symbols, and dose designations that are prone to misinterpretation and can result in prescription errors. The aforementioned list may be located at this location. An instance of potential confusion arises when the letter 'U' is mistakenly identified as the numerals '0' or '4'. This misinterpretation might lead to a significant tenfold escalation in the prescribed dose, particularly if the intention was to denote units. Consequently, it is highly recommended that the letter 'U' be substituted with the term 'units'.

Proficiency in medical abbreviations may be achieved via systematic study and regular practice. However, it is important to note that these abbreviations may first provide a significant challenge within the context of medical language. It is important to note that the aim is not to acquire knowledge of every abbreviation in existence, but rather to understand and effectively utilize those that are most pertinent to one's professional endeavors. This skill set will not only contribute to enhanced professional success in the field of medical coding, but it will also augment overall medical knowledge and facilitate more efficient navigation of the healthcare sector.

It is important to bear in mind that the comprehension of medical abbreviations encompasses more than the rote memorizing of a compendium of shorthand notations. Having a comprehensive understanding of the terminology employed in the medical domain and the ability to communicate effectively and succinctly, particularly in demanding circumstances, are crucial aspects to consider. Hence, equip yourself with this essential skill, and you will be one step closer to attaining success in your medical coding examination and progressing to the subsequent stage in your healthcare career.

Book 2: Anatomy & Physiology

Anatomy and Physiology by Body System

As one delves further into the human anatomy, a complex and interdependent network of systems is revealed, functioning in seamless coordination. A comprehensive understanding of the intricacies of the many physiological systems is crucial for individuals pursuing a successful career in the healthcare sector, especially for those engaged in medical coding and billing.

The exploration of the human body may be made less daunting by dividing it into its constituent systems and emphasizing key components and their respective functions.

This pertains to the physiological system responsible for the transportation of blood throughout the human body.

The circulatory system, often known as the cardiovascular system, is responsible for the transportation of blood, oxygen, and nutrition throughout the different regions of the body. The heart is a contractile organ responsible for the circulation of blood throughout the human body. The entity in question is often regarded as the central component of this particular system. The circulatory system comprises an intricate network of blood vessels, encompassing arteries, veins, and capillaries, which collectively facilitate the transportation of blood throughout the entirety of the human body.

The physiological mechanism accountable for the process of respiration

The gaseous exchange is facilitated by the circulatory system, which operates in coordination with the respiratory system to provide a mutually beneficial outcome. The respiratory system encompasses several anatomical structures, including the nasal cavity, pharynx, larynx, trachea, bronchi, and lungs. Simultaneously with the expulsion of carbon dioxide, which is a metabolic byproduct, the inhalation of oxygen occurs through the lungs and is then transported into the circulation.

This pertains to the anatomical system responsible for the breakdown, absorption, and assimilation of nutrients, also known as the digestive system.

The digestive system, spanning from the oral cavity through the intestines and terminating at the colon, is accountable for the conversion of ingested food into essential nutrients that can be utilized by the body. The human digestive system consists of several anatomical components, including the mouth cavity, esophagus, stomach, small intestine, large intestine, rectum, and anus. Additionally, this system is complemented by the presence and functions of the liver, gallbladder, and pancreas.

This pertains to the neurological system.

The nervous system functions as both the central regulatory and coordinating system, as well as the primary means of intercellular communication inside the human body. The human nervous system is comprised of three main components: the cranial region, the spinal cord, and the peripheral nerves that extend to the body's limbs. The central nervous system is responsible for the regulation and coordination of various bodily functions, encompassing activities such as heart rate, digestion, emotional experiences, and memory processes.

The musculoskeletal anatomy system

The network responsible for providing structural integrity and support to the body encompasses not just the skeletal system, but also the muscular system, tendons, and ligaments. Moreover, it serves to protect vital organs and facilitate bodily mobility. The facilitation of movement is facilitated by the muscular system, while the provision of structural support is attributed to the skeletal system.

This pertains to the urinary system.

The urinary system, often known as the renal system, comprises the kidneys, ureters, bladder, and urethra. The process of urine production is responsible for the removal of waste products from the body.

The biological mechanism accountable for the process of reproduction

The human reproductive process is regulated by this physiological system. The female reproductive system comprises the ovaries, fallopian tubes, uterus, and vagina. The male reproductive system consists of the testes, seminal vesicles, prostate gland, and penis.

The endocrine gland system

The endocrine system consists of a group of glands that are accountable for the production and release of hormones. Hormones are bioactive substances that serve as signaling molecules to regulate a diverse range of physiological processes within the body. Alongside many other glands, the endocrine system encompasses the pituitary gland, the thyroid gland, the adrenal glands, and the pancreas.

The term used to denote this physiological system is often known as the "Integumentary System."

The integumentary system, comprising the skin, hair, and nails, serves as a protective barrier against environmental harm inflicted upon the body. Furthermore, it contributes to the perception and regulation of temperature.

When delving further into each system, it is important to maintain a concentrated focus on the fundamental structures and their respective functions. Develop a comprehensive comprehension of the specialized terminology associated with each system, as well as the manner in which the constituent elements of each system mutually influence and engage with one another. The competence in reading medical information and associated coding techniques is valuable in this context.

This study aims to explore the prevailing issues, diagnostic approaches, and therapeutic interventions associated with various physiological systems, with the objective of enhancing our comprehensive comprehension of these systems. The possession of this information has significant importance for medical coders and billers as it enables them to have a more comprehensive understanding of the medical data they handle.

This pertains to the physiological mechanism responsible for the circulation of blood throughout the human body.

In conjunction with myocardial infarction, prevalent conditions affecting the circulatory system encompass hypertension and atherosclerosis. Hypertension, colloquially referred to as high blood pressure, and atherosclerosis, often known as hardening of the arteries, are among the notable illnesses in this domain. The electrocardiogram (ECG) is a diagnostic procedure utilized to assess the electrical impulses generated by the heart, whereas an angiogram is a diagnostic technique employed to see the arterial blood vessels. Both of these tests are conducted as part of diagnostic procedures. One potential therapeutic option for managing blood pressure is the administration of medication. However, individuals may also experience favorable outcomes by undergoing surgical interventions, such as angioplasty or bypass surgery.

The physiological mechanism accountable for the process of respiration

Several respiratory disorders, such as asthma, pneumonia, and chronic obstructive pulmonary disease (COPD), are recognized for their effects on the respiratory system. Both spirometry, a technique used to assess lung capacity, and bronchoscopy, a treatment that visually examines the airways, are considered diagnostic methods. The selection of treatments can differ according on the specific medical issue being addressed, encompassing the use of inhalers for asthma management and the administration of drugs for pneumonia.

This pertains to the anatomical system responsible for the breakdown and absorption of nutrients, often known as the digestive system.

Various diseases, including gastroesophageal reflux disease (GERD), commonly referred to as acid reflux, peptic ulcer disease, and colorectal cancer, have the potential to impact the functioning of the digestive system. Both endoscopy, a treatment that examines the digestive tract, and colonoscopy, a procedure that focuses on the colon, are diagnostic techniques that may be employed. The treatments for various ailments might vary significantly, encompassing a wide range of interventions. For instance, gastroesophageal reflux disease (GERD) may be managed with antacids, whereas colon cancer may necessitate surgical intervention.

This pertains to the neurological system.

Multiple sclerosis, Parkinson's disease, and stroke are representative instances of pathological conditions that have the potential to impact the functioning of the nervous system. Electroencephalography (EEG) and magnetic resonance imaging (MRI) are two diagnostic modalities employed for the assessment of cerebral electrical activity. Magnetic Resonance Imaging (MRI) has the capability to provide detailed visual representations of the brain and spinal cord, whilst Electroencephalography (EEG) is a technique used to quantify and analyze electrical activity inside same neural structures. The selection of treatment modalities is frequently customized to suit the specific medical state of each patient, encompassing potential interventions such as pharmacotherapy, rehabilitation, and in some cases, surgical procedures.

The musculoskeletal anatomy system

Fractures, osteoporosis, and rheumatoid arthritis are examples of illnesses that might potentially affect this physiological system. Radiographic imaging is employed to assess the skeletal structure and articulations, while bone densitometry scans are conducted to evaluate the presence of osteoporosis. Both of these procedures are diagnostic in nature. Potential therapeutic options for pain management include the utilization of various interventions such as physiotherapy and, in certain cases, surgical procedures.

This pertains to the urinary system.

Urinary tract infections, commonly referred to as UTIs, kidney stones, and chronic kidney disease are prevalent kidney illnesses frequently seen in clinical practice. Urinalysis, a diagnostic method that examines the constituents of urine, and ultrasonography, a diagnostic procedure that provides visual representation of the kidneys and bladder, are both often employed in clinical settings. Urinary tract infections (UTIs) are frequently treated with antibiotics, however in cases of renal impairment, dialysis is typically necessary.

The biological mechanism accountable for the process of reproduction

Various conditions can be observed in individuals, such as polycystic ovarian syndrome (PCOS) in females, erectile dysfunction in males, and sexually transmitted infections (STIs) in both genders. Polycystic ovary syndrome (PCOS) is a medical disorder characterized by its impact on the ovaries. Both an ultrasound of the female reproductive organs and an analysis of a sperm sample obtained from the male patient are considered diagnostic procedures. The management of polycystic ovary syndrome (PCOS) often encompasses the administration of hormone prescription, whereas the treatment of sexually transmitted infections (STIs) often necessitates the use of antibiotics.

The endocrine gland system

Conditions such as diabetes, hypothyroidism, and Addison's disease exemplify ailments that have the potential to impair the functionality of the endocrine system. Blood tests are commonly employed in diagnostic procedures to assess hormone levels. The management of various medical disorders typically involves the regulation of hormone levels, such as insulin in the context of diabetes.

The term used to denote this bodily system is often known as the "Integumentary System."

Acne, psoriasis, and skin cancer represent a subset of prevalent dermatological conditions. The spectrum of treatments for skin diseases include a variety of interventions, ranging from the use of topical creams to address acne and psoriasis, to the implementation of surgical procedures for the treatment of skin cancer. Biopsies, a diagnostic technique, can be employed for the examination of skin tissue.

The preservation of homeostasis is a fundamental aspect of human physiology. Homeostasis refers to the physiological process by which an organism maintains a stable internal environment, regardless of variations in external conditions or levels of physical exertion. The phenomenon being referred to is commonly recognized as homeostasis. The maintenance of this balance is crucial for the ongoing survival and optimal operation of the organism.

Every system inside the human body plays a vital role in maintaining homeostasis. The respiratory system is accountable for the regulation of oxygen and carbon dioxide levels in the bloodstream, whilst the circulatory system is responsible for the distribution of heat throughout the body to maintain a stable body temperature. The neurological and endocrine systems work as regulatory systems, whereby they provide signals to other physiological systems, instructing them to adapt their functioning in response to the body's internal conditions.

A comprehensive comprehension of homeostasis is crucial for anyone engaged in medical coding due to the significant association between several medical illnesses and the disruption of homeostatic mechanisms. For example, diabetes is a medical disorder characterized by the inability of the body to maintain homeostatic regulation of blood sugar levels. Various therapeutic approaches aim to restore homeostasis, including the use of insulin to regulate blood glucose levels in those afflicted with diabetes.

Now, let us transition to the subsequent subject matter and engage in a discussion pertaining to anatomical nomenclature. A comprehensive understanding of anatomical terminology is essential in effectively describing the many components and structures of the human body. The aforementioned terms has etymological roots in Latin or Greek and are widely acknowledged and routinely employed within the entirety of the medical discipline. Several terms are employed to describe the relative positioning of bodily structures. For instance, the term "anterior" denotes the front, "posterior" refers to the back, "superior" indicates a position above, "inferior" signifies a position below, "medial" denotes a direction toward the midline, and "lateral" signifies a direction away from the midline.

In the domain of medical coding, possessing a comprehensive understanding of anatomical terminology and employing it with precision has significant significance. The utilization of this particular linguistic framework is seen within medical documentation for the purpose of denoting the specific places of injuries, surgical interventions, or the sources of pathological conditions, all of which necessitate accurate and detailed descriptions. Additionally, it can be employed to delineate the geographical sites where surgical interventions are performed.

Finally, it is imperative to discuss the significance of the International Classification of Diseases (ICD) system. The International Classification of Diseases (ICD) is a universally adopted standardized coding system utilized for the classification of diseases and various health conditions on a global scale. This system enables the collection, analysis, interpretation, and comparison of health data. In the United States, medical coders utilize the ICD-10-CM (Clinical Modification) handbook for the purpose of diagnostic coding.

A comprehensive comprehension of the International Classification of Diseases (ICD) system is imperative for medical coders due to its predominant utilization within their professional responsibilities. It is employed in the practice of diagnostic coding throughout the whole healthcare sector, spanning from outpatient clinics to hospitals. Accurate documentation of patient diagnoses is vital for the purposes of invoicing, as well as for research and the compilation of health data. The assurance of this is achieved by the appropriate utilization of ICD coding.

A comprehensive grasp of the many physiological systems of the human body, the concept of homeostasis, the standardized anatomical terminology, and proficiency in utilizing the International Classification of Diseases (ICD) system are all fundamental prerequisites for achieving proficiency in the field of medical coding. Due to your acquired proficiency, you will possess the capability to proficiently interpret and encode medical records, hence facilitating the delivery of superior healthcare services to patients, ensuring precise financial transactions, and fostering advantageous advancements in health-related research. In order to achieve proficiency and efficiency in coding as a medical coder or biller, it is necessary to possess a comprehensive understanding of the human body's many systems, their functioning mechanisms, and the contextual factors that may impact these systems. The utilization of accurate coding practices contributes to effective billing procedures and informed medical decision-making, hence enhancing productivity and ultimately improving the overall quality of patient care. A comprehensive understanding of anatomy and physiology is essential in the subject of medical coding, as it encompasses more than just academic interest. A comprehensive understanding of the physiological systems of the human body, the many pathological illnesses that might potentially influence these systems, and the methodologies employed for the identification and management of these disorders is important in order to ensure precise coding. Hence, it is essential to bear in mind that embarking on one's academic journey entails more than just acquisition of factual knowledge. Instead, it involves cultivating a deep understanding of the intricate nature of the human body and its remarkable intricacies. The information offered here will considerably enhance the effectiveness of your medical coding profession by equipping you with the essential tools required for accurate and efficient coding.

Specific Coding-Related Anatomy

A fundamental requirement for accurate medical coding is an in-depth knowledge of the anatomy of the human body. Because of this expertise, it is possible to correctly understand the notes written by the physicians, which in turn assures appropriate coding and billing. When it comes to medical coding, it's important to zero in on the portions of the body that come up the most frequently. However, the human body is incredibly complex. This chapter will provide a road for newcomers to traverse this important component of their new career by delving into the essential anatomical ideas connected to medical coding. These topics will be covered in depth.

The Anatomy of the Circulatory System is presented here.

The cardiovascular system is another name for the circulatory system, which is made up of the heart and all of the blood vessels in the body, including the arteries, veins, and capillaries. Coders in the medical industry frequently come across terminology connected to this system, such as "myocardial infarction" (also known as "heart attack"), "angina pectoris" (also known as "chest pain"), and "peripheral arterial disease" (also known as "blocked arteries in the limbs").

A Dissection of the Anatomy of the Respiratory System

Inhaling oxygen and exhaling carbon dioxide are both part of the process of gas exchange, which is facilitated by the respiratory system, which consists of the nose, pharynx, larynx, trachea, bronchi, and lungs. The terms "pneumonia" (an infection of the lungs), "chronic obstructive pulmonary disease" (a long-term condition of the lungs), and "asthma" (a chronic inflammation of the airways) are frequently seen in the context of this system.

A Dissection of the Anatomy of the Digestive System

The digestive system, which extends from the mouth to the anus, is responsible for breaking down food into nutrients that may be absorbed. It is comprised of the esophagus, stomach, small intestine, and large intestine, in addition to auxiliary organs such as the gallbladder, pancreas, and liver. Coders in the medical industry commonly come across terminology like "gastritis" (which refers to inflammation of the stomach), "cholecystitis" (which refers to inflammation of the gallbladder), and "colitis" (which refers to inflammation of the colon).

The Nervous System's Anatomy and Physiology

The brain, spinal cord, and nerves throughout the body are all part of the nervous system, which is responsible for coordinating all of the body's operations. It is vital to have a working knowledge of words relating to neurological diseases. Some examples of these terms are "cerebrovascular accident" (also known as a stroke) and "multiple sclerosis" (a disease that damages nerve cells).

The structure and function of the musculoskeletal system

The musculoskeletal system is responsible for providing structure as well as the ability to move. It is composed of bones, muscles, joints, tendons, and ligaments. Coders in the medical industry frequently deal with diagnoses like "osteoarthritis," which refers to the deterioration of joint cartilage; "osteoporosis," which refers to the weakening of bones; and "fractures," which refers to fractured bones.

The genitourinary and reproductive systems are dissected in this anatomy lesson.

Urine is the means through which the urinary system, which includes the kidneys, ureters, bladder, and urethra, rids the body of waste materials. The human reproductive system consists of the testes, seminal vesicles, and penis in men and the ovaries, uterus, and vagina in females. This system is responsible for human reproduction and varies depending on the gender of the individual. Common names for this condition include "nephritis," which refers to inflammation of the kidneys; "cystitis," which refers to inflammation of the bladder; and "endometriosis," which refers to the development of uterine tissue outside of the uterus.

A Dissection of the Anatomy of the Endocrine System

Pituitary gland, thyroid gland, adrenal glands, and pancreas are examples of glands that are a part of the endocrine system. These glands are responsible for the production of hormones. Conditions such as "diabetes mellitus" (also known as excessive blood sugar) and "hyperthyroidism" (also known as an overactive thyroid gland) are associated with this system.

A Dissection of the Integumentary System

The integumentary system is a protective barrier that includes the skin, hair, and nails. Its function is to keep foreign substances out of the body. Coders frequently come across phrases like "dermatitis" (which refers to inflammation of the skin), "cellulitis" (which refers to an infection of the skin), and "melanoma" (which refers to cancer of the skin).

Keep in mind that proper coding is predicated on having a solid grasp of these biological systems and the parts that make them up. Make sure that your code always accurately represents the real nature of a patient's illness by always referring back to your grasp of anatomy as you progress through your coding career.

Coders in the medical field need to be knowledgeable with anatomical planes and directional words, in addition to having a fundamental knowledge of the body's many systems. Anatomical planes include the sagittal plane, the coronal plane, and the transverse plane. The sagittal plane divides the body into left and right, while the coronal plane divides the body into front and rear. The transverse plane divides the body into upper and lower. When describing the relative placement of different regions of the body, directional terminology such as anterior, posterior, superior, inferior, medial, and lateral are typically utilized.

Let's wrap this off with discussing the idea of bodily cavities, which is yet another critical component of comprehending human anatomy. The dorsal cavity (also known as the back side) and the ventral cavity (also known as the front side) are the two primary cavities that make up the body. Every one of them can be further subdivided into smaller cavities, which are home to a variety of organs. For instance, the abdominal cavity, which contains the digestive system, the urinary system, and the reproductive organs, and the thoracic cavity, which contains the heart and the lungs, are both included in the ventral cavity.

Your ability to correctly analyze and code medical data will be significantly improved if you have a more in-depth grasp of these anatomical principles. Your coding selections will be guided by this knowledge, and you will be able to give the most correct information for patient care, billing, and health statistics.

Some Useful Suggestions for Newcomers

1. Make consistent efforts to study anatomy: As a novice, it is essential to set aside regular study time in order to acquire an understanding of the anatomy of the human body. You may acquaint yourself with the various bodily systems by reading textbooks, using internet resources, or downloading anatomy applications.

2. Run Through Some Coding Scenarios for Practice: Put your understanding of anatomy to use by practicing different coding scenarios. You should now have a better understanding of how knowledge of anatomy pertains to coding in the real world.

3. Make some flashcards with the following: Create flashcards with common medical terminology that are relevant to each of the body's systems. Include the word, an explanation of the term, as well as an example of how the phrase may look in a medical record.

4. Make Use of [[Visual Aids]]: Understanding complicated anatomical structures may be made much easier with the use of visual aids like as diagrams and 3D models.

5. Think About Joining a Study Group: If you are interested in medical coding, you might think about joining a study group with other students. This might present possibilities to learn from other people, as well as to ask questions of them and obtain alternative viewpoints.

6. Inquire Concerning Don't be afraid to ask questions if you have any doubts about anything. Get in touch with your teachers or coworkers, or consult internet discussion groups, if you have any questions.

As you begin your journey into the realm of medical coding, keep in mind that being knowledgeable in the anatomy that is relevant to coding is a process that takes time. It is not necessary for you to grasp everything right now. Building a solid foundation in anatomy will take some time, patience, and constant study on your part, but in the long run, it will be beneficial to your future in medical coding.

Anatomy of the Heart and the Diseases of the Cardiovascular System

The muscular organ known as the heart is responsible for pumping blood through the circulatory system. It has two atria at the top and two ventricles at the bottom, making a total of four primary chambers in its structure. In addition to these chambers, the heart contains four valves that control the flow of blood both within the heart and to the rest of the body.

When working in medical coding, you will frequently come across cardiovascular disorders. These disorders include coronary artery disease, in which the arteries that supply the heart muscle become narrowed or clogged, which can lead to chest discomfort (also known as angina) or a heart attack (also known as a myocardial infarction). Heart failure is another prevalent ailment. This occurs when the heart is unable to pump blood adequately, which results in symptoms such as shortness of breath and fluid retention. Heart failure may be prevented by maintaining a healthy blood pressure.

The Anatomy of the Lungs and the Diseases that Affect the Respiratory System

The lungs are the primary organs of the respiratory system. They are responsible for drawing oxygen into the body while simultaneously expelling carbon dioxide. There are lobes in both the right and left lungs, with three lobes in the right lung and two in the left lung respectively. The bronchi inside the lungs branch off into even smaller tubes called bronchioles, which ultimately terminate in alveoli, the microscopic air sacs that are the sites of gas exchange.

When working in medical coding, you will frequently come across respiratory disorders such as chronic obstructive pulmonary disease (COPD). COPD is an umbrella term that refers to a group of ailments that can make it difficult to breathe, including emphysema and chronic bronchitis. Asthma is another prevalent ailment that causes wheezing, shortness of breath, and coughing in patients. It is a chronic inflammatory disease that causes the airways to become more constricted.

The Structure of the Brain and Its Relation to Neurological Conditions

The brain is the primary organ of the nervous system and is composed of a number of distinct regions, each of which is accountable for a certain set of activities. These include the cerebrum, which is in charge of higher processes like as intellect and action, the cerebellum, which is in charge of movement coordination, and the brainstem, which is in charge of fundamental activities such as the rate at which you breathe and your heartbeat.

Neurological illnesses are diseases that affect the nervous system, which includes the brain and spinal cord. Alzheimer's disease is a degenerative ailment that causes brain cells to waste away and die, leading to memory loss and cognitive decline. Other common disorders include stroke, in which blood supply to part of the brain is cut off, causing brain cells to die; and multiple sclerosis, in which the body's immune system attacks and destroys nerve cells.

The Anatomy of the Digestive Tract as well as Disorders of the Gastrointestinal Tract

The digestive process begins in the mouth and continues all the way down to the anus. The esophagus, stomach, and small and large intestines are located in the middle of the digestive tract. The digestion of food, the absorption of nutrients, and the elimination of waste are all handled by separate sections of the digestive tract.

Conditions such as gastroesophageal reflux disease (GERD), in which acid from the stomach travels back into the esophagus, are included in the category of gastrointestinal diseases. GERD can cause heartburn and other symptoms. Inflammatory bowel disease (IBD), also known as Crohn's disease and ulcerative colitis, are both chronic inflammatory illnesses that affect the digestive tract. IBD is a prevalent ailment that affects many people.

Anatomy of the Musculoskeletal System and the Conditions of Orthopedics

Muscles and bones make up the musculoskeletal system, which also includes the joints, ligaments, and tendons that connect these structures to one another. This system not only facilitates mobility but also helps to sustain the structure of the body.

When working in the field of medical coding, one will commonly come across orthopedic disorders like fractures, which occur when a bone breaks as a result of an injury or disease. Osteoarthritis is another frequent ailment that causes pain and stiffness in the joints. It is a degenerative joint disease that arises when the protective cartilage that cushions the ends of your bones wears away over time, causing osteoarthritis to develop.

Anatomy of the Endocrine System as well as Disorders of the Endocrine System

The endocrine system is a network of glands that create and secrete hormones, which are responsible for regulating a wide variety of processes throughout the body. The pituitary gland, the thyroid gland, the parathyroid gland, the adrenal glands, the pancreas, the ovaries, and the testes are the key glands that make up the endocrine system.

When it comes to medical coding, endocrine problems are rather widespread. Diabetes mellitus is one of these conditions; it's a disease that's defined by excessive blood sugar levels owing to insulin resistance or lack of insulin production. Hypothyroidism is another prevalent ailment that can lead to symptoms such as fatigue, weight gain, and depression. This condition occurs when the thyroid gland does not generate sufficient amounts of the hormone thyroid.

Anatomy of the Urinary System as well as Disorders of the Urological System

Urine is the primary means through which the urinary system flushes waste items out of the body. It is comprised of the kidneys, which are responsible for filtering blood in order to generate urine, the ureters, which are tubes that transport urine from the kidneys to the bladder, the bladder, which is a sac that stores urine, and the urethra, which is a tube that transports pee from the bladder out of the body.

Urological conditions are also often seen in medical coding. Urinary tract infections are among them, which occur when bacteria enter the urinary tract and cause infection. This infection can frequently result in symptoms such as discomfort and the need to urinate frequently. Kidney stones are another frequent ailment that may cause excruciating pain. Kidney stones are hard deposits formed of minerals and salts that occur inside your kidneys and can develop at any time.

Anatomy of the Reproductive System as well as Disorders of the Reproductive System

The reproductive system is the organ that's in charge of reproduction in humans. This system consists of the testes, the prostate gland, and the penis in males. Testes are responsible for the production of sperm. In females, it is composed of the ovaries, the uterus, and the vagina. Ovaries are responsible for egg production.

In the field of medical coding, reproductive diseases are encountered often. In women, this can manifest as illnesses such as polycystic ovarian syndrome (PCOS), which is characterized by an imbalance in the production of hormones that results in the development of tiny cysts on the ovaries. This can lead to symptoms such as irregular periods and infertility. In males, illnesses such as prostate enlargement or prostate cancer are frequent disorders that can produce symptoms such as difficulty urinating and pelvic discomfort.

Anatomy of the Integumentary System and Conditions Related to Dermatology

The skin, hair, and nails, as well as the glands that produce perspiration and oil, are all components of the integumentary system. It acts as a barrier between the body and the outside world, providing protection for the body.

In clinical settings, dermatological problems are typically classified as diagnoses. Psoriasis is an example of one of these disorders. Psoriasis is a skin ailment that causes skin cells to proliferate up to ten times faster than they normally would. This results in red areas that are rough and are covered with white scales. Atopic dermatitis, more often known as eczema, is another frequent disorder that causes redness and itching of the skin.

Medical coders may assure the appropriate translation of medical information into codes by first gaining an awareness of the architecture of these body systems and the major disorders that affect them. Your job in medical coding will benefit greatly from the combination of this information, ongoing training and practice, and continued education. It is absolutely necessary for correct medical coding to have an understanding of the architecture of various biological systems as well as the illnesses that might impact them. Your knowledge may be increased over time through the combination of regular study and practice. Do not forget to make use of resources such as anatomy textbooks and internet resources, and do not be afraid to ask questions if something is confusing. Your commitment to gaining knowledge about, and having a comprehension of, anatomy will serve you well as you pursue a career in medical coding.

When it comes to medical coding, having a strong grasp of anatomy is essential; nevertheless, it is also necessary to be aware of the potential ethical difficulties that may arise in the field. Coders in the medical industry frequently face challenges that need them to meet ethical norms. There may be pressure, for instance, to up code or down code in order to maximize reimbursement or lower the expenses incurred by patients. In times like these, it is absolutely necessary to maintain a firm stance and act in accordance with the Code of Ethics established by the American Health Information Management Association (AHIMA). Not only does upholding these ethical principles safeguard patients, but it also ensures that the confidentiality of health information is preserved. You will be well-prepared to achieve success in the field of medical coding if you demonstrate this dedication to ethical conduct and possess a thorough grasp of anatomy.

Book 3: CPT, HCPCS, and ICD-10 Coding

Introduction to the CPT Coding System

Coding according to CPT, often known as Current Procedural Terminology, is an essential part of the healthcare industry. It is a vocabulary system that is defined and utilized throughout the United States to describe the numerous services and operations that are carried out by healthcare practitioners. These codes are essential for billing, record keeping, and data analysis. They provide consistency and accuracy in the manner in which medical services are reported and compensated.

Comprehending the CPT Coding System

The American Medical Association (AMA) is the organization responsible for the development and administration of CPT codes. They may be broken down into the following three categories:

1. In "Category I," we have: These are numeric numbers with a length of five digits that correspond to treatments that are often carried out by medical professionals. They span a broad spectrum of services, including as evaluation and management (E&M) services, imaging services, and surgical operations.

2. "In the second category:" These are tracking numbers consisting of alphanumeric that are used for performance evaluation. They are not necessary, but the additional data they give regarding the care's quality might be useful.

3. In "Category III," which is: These are ephemeral alphanumeric codes that are put into use for developing practices and services that are still in the testing phase.

The Significance of CPT Coding in Healthcare

CPT codes are extremely important in the following areas of the healthcare industry:

- Reimbursement and Billing: They ensure that the reporting of services rendered is standardized, which gives insurance carriers the ability to comprehend the costs of treatments and appropriately recoup those costs.

- Analyzing the Data and Doing Some Research: The creation of a consistent language for procedures is one of the many contributions that the Current

Procedural Terminology (CPT) coding system makes to the advancement of research and policy.

CPT codes are able to assist in tracking the success of medical therapies, which contributes to performance assessment and improvement.

Helpful Hints for Getting Started with CPT Coding

The world of CPT coding may appear to be complicated when you are just starting out, but there are ways that can make the process of learning it easier:

- Make the Investment in an Up-to-Date CPT Code Book: This ought to serve as your major source of reference. Because the AMA makes changes to it on a yearly basis, you need to be sure you have the most recent copy.

- Get Familiar with the Organization of the CPT Code Book: Become knowledgeable about the structure of the book and how it is laid out. It is organized into parts that pertain to the various bodily systems as well as the many medical specializations.

- Practice Making Use of Modifiers: In order to offer more information about an operation, CPT codes can be supplemented by two-digit codes known as modifiers.

- Make Regular Practices: As with learning any new ability, the more you put in the effort to practice, the more at ease you will feel. To evaluate your level of understanding, you can use practice tasks and quizzes.

- Become a Member of a Professional Organization: Learning, networking, and professional certification are all available through the tools provided by organizations such as the American Academy of Professional Coders (AAPC).

The Most Frequent Problems With CPT Coding

It's possible that you'll run into a few obstacles while you learn CPT coding, but you shouldn't let that deter you. Having an awareness of these typical challenges might assist you in overcoming them:

- Adapting to New Developments: Because the CPT codes are revised on an annual basis, maintaining a current knowledge base demands continuous education.

Acquiring an Understanding of Medical Terminology: It is absolutely necessary to have a strong foundation in medical language in order to comprehend and properly use CPT codes.

Managing Complicated Matter and Precise Information: There are certain operations that may be coded in numerous ways, depending on the specific conditions. The acquisition of the skills necessary to negotiate these complexities requires time and practice.

It is impossible to express how vitally important it is to have proper CPT coding in the field of telemedicine. The demand for accurate coding of remote healthcare services is growing in tandem with the expansion of these services themselves. When reporting patient contacts that take place through the use of telecommunications technology, telemedicine makes use of a particular set of CPT codes. Another crucial component of being an expert in CPT coding is becoming familiar with these codes.

Methods for Deciphering CPT Codes

Each and every CPT code is one of a kind and can contain a plethora of information. Deciphering the meaning of a CPT code requires first having a solid understanding of its structure.

- "The first digit" denotes the category of the CPT code, with "1" indicating Category I, "0" indicating Category II, and "G" or "T" indicating Category III.

The next four digits contain information that is more detailed about the process or service that will be performed.

For instance, the first number of the CPT code 99213 is a "9," which indicates that the code belongs to Category I, while the other digits, "9213," offer specifics on the kind of service that was rendered.

Coding Guidelines for the CPT

The American Medical Association (AMA) releases recommendations that might assist coders in making appropriate use of CPT codes. These rules explain how to select the appropriate code for an operation or service, as well as how to apply modifiers and other crucial information. It is absolutely necessary to stay current with these rules in order to keep the correctness of the coding in check.

Comparison of CPT Codes, ICD Codes, and HCPCS Codes

Although they are extremely important, CPT codes are not the only type of coding utilized in the healthcare industry. The International Classification of Diseases (ICD) codes, which are used to define patient diagnoses, and the Healthcare Common Procedure Coding System (HCPCS) codes, which include services and procedures that are not included in the CPT system, are frequently used in combination with the CPT codes. The key to successful comprehensive medical coding is having a solid understanding of the distinctions and connections between different systems.

CPT Coding Should Take Into Account Ethical Considerations

The field of medical coding places a substantial emphasis on ethical considerations. Coders have the responsibility of ensuring that they pick the most correct codes possible to reflect the services that were rendered, taking care not to over code (which can result in fraudulent claims and legal concerns) or under code (which might lead to insufficient compensation). It is absolutely necessary, in order to keep the reliability of the healthcare system intact, to be aware of these ethical problems.

The Importance of Receiving Proper Certification When CPT Coding

Certification is a useful tool for demonstrating your competence in CPT coding, however it is not always necessary. Exams for certification in medical coding are made available by groups such as the American Academy of Professional Coders (AAPC) and the American Health Information Management Association (AHIMA). Acquiring one or more of these credentials can raise your level of credibility, broaden your employment opportunities, and possibly result in a higher salary.

The Prospects for the CPT Coding System

The field of CPT coding, much like the healthcare industry as a whole, is in a state of perpetual evolution. On a regular basis, new codes are introduced in order to accurately represent newly developed processes and technologies, while older codes are removed. In addition, the move toward digital health records and computerized coding systems is altering the landscape of the medical profession. In order to achieve success in the field of medical coding, it will be necessary to have a flexible mindset and be current with these developments.

Medical Specialties and the CPT Coding System

CPT codes are utilized in a variety of medical subspecialties and fields. Learning the CPT codes that are particular to your area of expertise might help you work more quickly and accurately. The CPT code book is divided into separate parts for each medical specialty. For instance, cardiology has its own unique set of codes for procedures such as echocardiograms and angioplasties, whereas psychiatry has its own unique set of codes for services such as psychotherapy and mental diagnostic evaluations.

Services Regarding CPT Coding and E/M Exams

The provision of evaluation and management services, sometimes known as E/M services, is an important component of medical treatment. The medical state of the patient is evaluated, and appropriate treatment and care are provided. The coding of E/M services follows its own unique set of guidelines, which take into consideration a variety of aspects, including the degree of difficulty involved in making a medical decision and the amount of time spent with the patient. The E/M coding system underwent considerable revisions in 2021, which made it absolutely necessary for coders to remain up to speed and comprehend the modifications.

Errors in CPT Coding: Their Consequences and How to Avoid Them

Errors in CPT coding have the potential to have major ramifications, including inaccurate billing, claims that are delayed or refused, possible audits, and legal penalties. Therefore, it is absolutely necessary to steer clear of typical errors such as:

Which Is Better: Upcoding or Down coding? This refers to coding for a greater or lower quality of service than what was actually given. It can happen either intentionally or unintentionally. It is very necessary to code for the service that is documented in the health record of the patient at all times.

- Decoupling: This situation arises when various codes are used to record services that need to be reported under a single code that encompasses them all. In order to avoid this, you should become familiar with the coding rules and the idea of using "global packages" in certain processes.

Incorrect Use of Modifiers: Although modifiers offer extra information on a service or procedure, their use that is not accurate can lead to misunderstanding, which in turn can lead to incorrect invoicing.

It is crucial to have a comprehensive grasp of CPT codes, to remain current with changes in coding requirements, and to ensure that accurate and extensive documentation of patient contacts is maintained in order to avoid these mistakes.

The Importance of Technology in the CPT Coding Process

The landscape of CPT coding is undergoing change as a result of the introduction of electronic health records (EHR) and coding technologies powered by artificial intelligence. These technologies can help automate the coding process, which will cut down on errors caused by human labor and improve overall productivity. However, this does not eliminate the necessity for highly competent coding professionals. Coders are still need to inspect and validate the code that is produced by these tools in order to guarantee that it is correct.

In light of the current COVID-19 epidemic, the significance of CPT coding that is both correct and up to date has come under increased scrutiny. The American

Medical Association (AMA) has developed a number of new CPT codes in order to account for the many different services that are associated with COVID-19. These services include testing, immunization, and telemedicine services. For the time being, it is essential for all CPT coders to stay updated on these changes and have a solid grasp of how to implement the newly released codes.

You are an integral component of a process that serves as the foundation of the medical care delivery system if you are a CPT coder. Your efforts will guarantee that medical services are represented accurately, which will, in turn, make billing, research, and policy-making more straightforward. Your job as a medical coder will continue to increase in significance and complexity as a result of the ongoing change in the healthcare industry, allowing you a career path that is both lucrative and demanding codes offer a method of recording and billing for services in the field of preventive medicine that are focused at preventing sickness or identifying it at an early stage. Immunizations, tests, and counseling services are all examples of what falls under this category. Another essential component of accurate CPT coding is having a solid grasp on how these procedures should be coded.

You, in your capacity as a medical coder, play an essential part in the financial well-being of your healthcare organization as well as the overarching mission of precisely documenting and assessing the quality of healthcare services. It is a duty that necessitates exactness, ongoing education, and a dedication to conducting business in an ethical manner. The field of CPT coding is one that is always changing and developing. Coding standards are always being updated to take into account the many developments that occur in the healthcare industry. Always keep your mind open to new information, never stop learning, and view obstacles as chances for personal development. When you decide to enter the field of CPT coding, you are not just making a career decision; you are also making a commitment to the ongoing improvement of the quality and delivery of healthcare.

Using the CPT Manual and Conventions

The Current Procedural Terminology (CPT) Manual serves as a comprehensive compendium that serves as a foundational resource for all those engaged in CPT coding. The issuance of this document is attributed to the American Medical Association (AMA). The book has a systematic organization and encompasses a multitude of codes aimed at establishing uniformity across diverse diagnostic, surgical, and medical interventions. Acquiring the requisite abilities to effectively navigate and utilize the CPT coding manual is crucial for achieving success in this domain.

A Comprehensive Examination of the Structural Framework of the Current Procedural Terminology (CPT) Manual

The CPT manual is composed of three separate components, which are outlined as follows:

In the category labeled as "Category I," the following items are included: This particular domain is quite extensive, encompassing a wide range of codes pertaining to various operations and services that are well recognized and accepted within the professional medical community.

In the second category, there are alphabetic and numeric codes that are employed on a voluntary basis for the specific objectives of performance evaluation and data aggregation.

In the work titled "Category III," the following elements are presented: This section contains tentative codes for emerging technologies, services, and operational procedures.

Each of these components is further divided into subsections and subheadings, which are structured based on the physiological systems or specialized medical fields. It is advisable to acquaint oneself with these divisions in order to expedite the process of locating the required codes.

The requirements, guidelines, and conventions outlined in the CPT Manual.

The CPT manual has a series of recommendations that prescribe the appropriate utilization of codes. The guidelines encompass essential guidance pertaining to the selection of suitable code, the utilization of modifiers, and other pertinent information of significance. In order to maximize the accuracy of your code, it is imperative that you possess a comprehensive understanding of these regulations.

The guidebook furthermore employs certain conventions in order to provide additional information on the codes. Several instances of these standards encompass symbols, abbreviations, and punctuation. One example of the utilization of a semicolon in coding is to minimize space by indicating shared components between codes. Similarly, the adoption of a bullet symbol serves to indicate the introduction of a novel technique or service subsequent to the previous edition. Both of these symbols have been included in the current version, subsequent to the prior one.

Acquire Practical Knowledge by Utilizing the CPT Manual

One might enhance their familiarity with the CPT manual by engaging in practical exercises. To begin, select a number in a random manner, and thereafter search for that number inside the instructional handbook. One may also engage in the practical application of coding by working with authentic medical cases or sample medical records, so enhancing one's proficiency in this domain. The practical nature of this technique may aid in familiarizing oneself with the organization of the manual and developing comprehension of the coding procedure.

The incorporation of modifiers and appendices in academic writing

To provide more details on a medical procedure, CPT codes can be augmented by modifiers, which are two-character codes. The CPT guide has a comprehensive list of these modifiers, along with the corresponding regulations for their implementation.

The manual furthermore has several appendices with informative content that proves beneficial to the reader. Appendix A provides an extensive examination of modifiers, while Appendix B presents a summary of the revisions that have been implemented in the manual over the previous year.

Ensuring the Up-to-Date Edition of Your Current Procedural Terminology Manual

It is important to own a current edition of the CPT handbook due to its yearly revisions that align with evolving medical practices. Individuals will be provided with sufficient time to familiarize themselves with the alterations prior to their obligatory implementation, as the American Medical Association (AMA) typically adheres to the customary practice of releasing the updated version towards the latter of the year.

Understanding Various Coding Scenarios

It is conceivable that some activities or services may possess distinctive coding situations that want further understanding. For example, packaged codes consolidate many discrete yet interconnected services into a unified identification. The practice of unbundling these services or utilizing separate codes for each of them is considered to be incorrect coding. In order to effectively navigate unusual scenarios, it is imperative to possess a comprehensive awareness of the criteria outlined in the CPT handbook.

Given that we have previously covered the foundational principles of employing the CPT manual, let us now progress towards more advanced strategies and recommendations aimed at enhancing your proficiency in this domain.

An In-Depth Examination of Utilizing Tabular Lists and the Index

The CPT manual consists of two main components, namely the Alphabetic Index and the Tabular List.

The coding procedure will commence from this point onwards, as shown by the alphabetical index. The entity in question is a compilation of lexical units, systematically arranged in alphabetical order, accompanied by corresponding symbolic representations. Prior to implementing any code from the Tabular List, it is imperative to verify its accuracy.

- Table of Contents: This portion of the Current Procedural Terminology (CPT) manual serves as the main component, encompassing a comprehensive compilation of codes and corresponding guidelines dictating their appropriate utilization.

The enhancement of one's ability to swiftly transition between these two sections will result in a higher level of coding proficiency.

A Taxonomy of Comprehension for Programming Code

The CPT codes in the Tabular List are arranged in a specified pattern. For example, the initial code inside a given section or subsection frequently represents the service that is most comprehensive in scope, but subsequent codes offer services that are either more specific or supplemental in nature. Having a comprehensive comprehension of this hierarchical structure will facilitate the process of selecting the most accurate code for a certain service.

The appropriate utilization of punctuation and formatting

The CPT handbook has a specific punctuation and style scheme to effectively communicate information regarding the codes. Consider, for example:

The use of parentheses in text serves to provide more information on a code that is deemed nonessential.

The user's text should be revised to adhere to academic writing standards. No further information should be added.

Indentation is commonly employed when presenting a hierarchical structure of discrete activities that are subsumed inside a broader code.

Individuals who possess a comprehensive comprehension of these formatting rules should have no difficulties in appropriately comprehending the codes.

Employing Precise Instructions and Guidelines

The CPT manual provides instructions in many sections, each of which has specific coding rules applicable to that particular sector. Moreover, supplementary details pertaining to a specific code or a collection of codes may be accessed in the handbook by means of annotations, which are dispersed throughout the written material. It is crucial that you thoroughly read and interpret the included instructions and notes in order to ensure accurate coding. Therefore, it is strongly advised that you do so immediately.

The utilization of illustrations plays a crucial role in enhancing the effectiveness of conveying information.

The CPT manual has a comprehensive collection of anatomical photographs pertaining to a wide range of surgical procedures, prominently shown within its dedicated section. Visual aids may be highly beneficial for those who have a preference for visual learning, since they can greatly enhance their understanding of the essential aspects of a given process.

In order to stay current with the most recent information, it is essential to engage in continuous learning and remain abreast of the latest developments in one's field of interest. This may be achieved by several means, including as attending conferences, participating in professional development programs, subscribing to scholarly journals, and actively networking with experts in the field. By actively seeking out and assimilating new knowledge, individuals can enhance their

It is crucial to stay up-to-date with the updates of the CPT manual, considering its annual review cycle. The American Medical Association (AMA) provides a range of resources that can aid in understanding the modifications, including the CPT Changes publication and web-based instructional modules. By employing these tools, individuals may effectively maintain their coding proficiency and achieve success in their endeavors.

It is important to bear in mind that attaining proficiency in applying the CPT handbook is a skill that can solely be gained by practical experience. As one engages in continuous practice and gains expertise, their ability to accurately pick suitable codes and know the intricacies of the CPT coding system will improve. This will enable individuals to enhance their efficiency. It is imperative to maintain a continuous pursuit of knowledge acquisition and personal growth. In instances of encountering obstacles, it is essential to overcome any hesitations and seek assistance or clarification. The level of commitment exhibited towards acquiring expertise in the CPT manual will significantly impact the degree of success achieved in the field of medical coding. In the current era characterized by swift technology progress, the process of perusing the CPT manual has become notably more accessible than in previous times. A considerable proportion of programmers already utilize digital versions of the manual, which offer benefits such as enhanced search capabilities and streamlined navigation. Acquiring proficiency in utilizing these digital tools will enhance one's programming capabilities in terms of efficiency and accuracy.

It is important to note that achieving proficiency in utilizing the CPT manual is a task that cannot be expedited. The endeavor necessitates a substantial investment of time, exertion, and tenacity. As individuals further familiarize themselves with the handbook and its norms, they will cultivate an enhanced sense of self-confidence and improve their coding proficiency. Becoming proficient in CPT coding may be achieved via consistent and dedicated work. This would enable individuals to actively participate in the crucial endeavor of accurately documenting and reporting healthcare services.

CPT Modifiers and Examples

The application of modifiers is one aspect of CPT coding that contributes to an additional layer of complexity while also enhancing precision. CPT codes can have two-character codes added to them called modifiers. These modifiers offer extra information about the service or treatment that was carried out. It is essential to have a solid understanding of how to apply modifiers appropriately in order to achieve accurate coding and maximized reimbursement.

An Introduction to the CPT Modifiers

CPT modifiers provide more information describing the treatment or service, changing or expanding the description to ensure that the particular conditions of the process are appropriately represented in the code. They may, among other things, include information regarding a number of different procedures that were carried out, services that were provided by more than one physician, or services that were carried out in various parts of the body.

Frequent CPT Modifiers and How to Apply Them

Let's take a look at some of the most popular CPT modifiers and the situations in which they are used:

The 24th Modifier says: During the postoperative phase, this modifier is applied to indicate that the same physician performed an evaluation and management service that was unrelated to the surgery.

The 25th Modifier says: This modifier is applied when reporting a substantial E/M service that can be identified individually and was performed on the same day as a procedure or other treatment by the same physician.

Modifier 50 : When reporting bilateral operations that are done during the same operating session by the same physician, this modifier should be used.

Modifier 51 : This modification is included to the report when more than one procedure was carried out on the same patient by the same doctor on the same day.

The 59th Modifier is as follows: This modifier is used to denote a distinct procedural service, indicating that the service is different and not a part of another procedure. This signifies that the service is separate and not a part of the procedure.

Some Illustrations of CPT Modifiers

Having several samples to look at makes it much easier to comprehend the appropriate utilization of modifiers. Here are several examples:

The following is an example of modifier 24: Let's say a patient underwent surgery, and then during the postoperative time, they went to the same physician for treatment of an unrelated ailment. What would happen? Following the E/M CPT code and then adding the 24 modifier would be the proper way to record the surgeon's evaluation and management service for that appointment.

The following is an example of modifier 25: The 25 modifier would be added to the E/M service code if a patient went to their doctor for a standard checkup (an E/M service), and while they were there, they also received a flu vaccine (a separate treatment). In this scenario, the patient's doctor would bill for both procedures separately.

Exemplification of the Modifier 50: The operation code would be followed by the 50 modifier in the event that a doctor performed a tonsillectomy on both sides (bilateral) during the same operating session.

Common Mistakes That Can Be Made With CPT Modifiers

Misuse of CPT modifiers can lead to improper coding and, in some cases, a claim being denied even when the modifiers themselves contain required data. The following are some typical hazards that you should try to avoid:

- Excessive Use of Modifiers: When the standard procedure code does not adequately convey the nature of the service being rendered, only then should modifiers be used. An excessive amount of utilization may result in increased attention from payers as well as potential audits.

- Erroneous Use of the Modifier: There is a purpose for each and every modifier, and if you apply the incorrect modifier, it might lead to mistakes in your coding. Before you use a modifier, check that you have a complete understanding of its function.

- In the Following Order: It is possible for the order to have an effect on the reimbursement when many modifiers are applied. In most cases, the modification that has the greatest potential to dramatically affect reimbursement need to be stated first.

Adapting to the Constant Changes

The standards for using CPT modifiers, as well as the list of CPT modifiers, are frequently updated. As a result, staying current with the most recent modifications made by the AMA is quite necessary. To guarantee that your coding is accurate at all times, you should routinely check and update your expertise.

Various Other CPT Modifiers and How to Apply Them

In addition to the typical modifiers that we covered previously, here are a few more frequent ones that you'll likely come across:

The 26th Modifier says: This modifier is used to indicate the professional component of a service or procedure that includes both professional and technical components. Examples of services and procedures that have both professional and technical components include.

The 32nd modifier says: When a service is required by parties other than the patient, like as insurance companies or government authorities, this modifier is applied to describe the situation.

The following is Modifier 57: Used to signify that the original decision to undertake surgery was brought about as a consequence of an Evaluation and Management (E/M) service.

The following is Modifier 91's commentary: When reporting results of repeated laboratory tests or studies carried out on the same day, this modifier should be used.

Additional Modifiers Shown Through Examples
Having examples at hand can make it much simpler to comprehend these extra modifiers:

The following is an example of modifier 26: Imagine that a radiologist is tasked with providing their interpretation of an x-ray that was obtained at a hospital. In order to show that they are only charging for the professional component (interpretation) of the service and not the technical component (taking the x-ray), the radiologist would submit the x-ray CPT code with the modifier 26. This would indicate that they are only invoicing for the professional component of the service.

The following is an example of modifier 32: It is necessary for the consulting physician to record the relevant E/M code together with the modifier 32 in the event that the patient's insurance company demands a second opinion prior to authorizing surgery.

The following is an example of modifier 57: After providing an E/M service, if a doctor thereafter decides to conduct major surgery on a patient, the E/M service code should be recorded with the modifier 57 attached to it.

The following is an example of modifier 91: If a laboratory retests a patient's sample on the same day to confirm original results, the retest would be recorded with the same code as the first test, but with the modifier 91 added. This is because the retest is considered a confirmation of the previous test.

Documentation's Role and Importance
The right application of modifiers is intricately intertwined with the documentation process. In the absence of evidence that is both comprehensive and correct, the utilization of a modifier may be called into doubt, which may result in the denial of a claim or in a delay in payment. As a result, it is very necessary to have documentation that is both clear and comprehensive and that explains the use of each modification.

The Function That Modifiers Play Within the E/M System
When it comes to developing E/M services, modifiers play a key role. The medical need of a service, the participation of other specialists, or the intricacy of medical decision-making are all examples of characteristics of E/M services that frequently require extra explanation. In situations like these, modifiers like 24, 25, and 57 are quite helpful, and they are utilized often in E/M code.

What Role Do Modifiers Play in the Reimbursement Process?
The influence that modifiers have on reimbursement can be considerable. Because the surgery is carried out on both sides of the body, for instance, the use of modifier 50, which denotes a "bilateral procedure," typically results in a reimbursement of 150%. In a similar vein, the use of modifier 51, which refers to "multiple procedures," typically results in a reduction in reimbursement for the secondary treatments. If you have a good understanding of these implications,

you will be better able to forecast how the application of a modifier will influence the reimbursement of a claim.

In conclusion, CPT modifiers are a very useful instrument in the hands of an experienced coder. You may prevent claims from being denied, ensuring that the coding is accurate, and make it easier for people to get reimbursed fairly if you appropriately apply these modifications. However, ongoing study and practice are essential if one wants to achieve mastery of modifiers. You will become increasingly skilled in the art of modifier application as you acquire experience and remain current with the most recent modifications. As a result, you will become an essential component of the process by which healthcare reimbursement is determined modifiers are vital in the ever-changing environment of the healthcare industry because of the high degree of detail they give. The correct portrayal of the clinical condition that modifiers make possible is what ultimately leads to equitable remuneration and efficient communication between healthcare providers and payers. You may dramatically improve the accuracy of your CPT coding and become a useful contributor to the healthcare coding system if you understand and appropriately apply modifiers to your codes. Modifiers can be found in the CPT manual.

Introduction to HCPCS Level II Coding

The maze-like nature of medical coding can be intimidating for those just starting out, but if one has a solid foundation of knowledge and is guided appropriately, the process can become substantially less difficult. The HCPCS Level II codes are an important component of this overall coding scheme. HCPCS is an acronym that stands for Healthcare Common Procedure Coding System. HCPCS (which is pronounced "hick-picks") is a standardized coding system that was designed by the Centers for Medicare and Medicaid Services (CMS). The HCPCS Level II codes are made up of letters and numbers, and its primary purpose is to identify non-physician services such as ambulance services, long-term medical equipment, and prostheses, amongst other things.

Having an Understanding of the HCPCS Level II Codes

The HCPCS Level II coding system is utilized in the healthcare industry for the purpose of reporting a wide variety of services and products. These codes are especially important to use when invoicing for patients who are covered by Medicare and Medicaid, but a wide variety of other insurers also demand their use. The HCPCS Level II coding system is segmented into series, with each series being denoted by a single alphabetic letter and then four digits of a numerical representation.

Organization of Codes Used in HCPCS Level II

The initial character of an HCPCS Level II code is a capital letter that can be any one of the letters A through V. This particular letter identifies the sequence to which the code belongs. Every series is organized to correspond to a certain kind of service or supply. Take, for example:

- The A-codes include things like travel, medical and surgical supplies, and various and experimental things.
- B-codes: Parenteral and Enteral Nutritional Support
Temporary Hospital Outpatient Prospective Payment System (C-codes) and Durable Medical Equipment (E-codes)
- J-codes: Drugs Administered Other Than Orally, and Drugs Used in Chemotherapy

The next four numbers, all of which are numeric, give more information about the product or service.

Application in Real-World Settings of HCPCS Level II Codes

Let's take a look at a real-world scenario to better understand how to apply HCPCS Level II codes. Take for example a patient who suffers from chronic obstructive pulmonary disease (COPD) and needs oxygen equipment that they may use at home. The provider of long-lasting medical equipment (DME) would submit their claims to Medicare using the number E0424, which stands for "Stationary Compressed Gaseous Oxygen System."

The Significant Role That Modifiers Play in HCPCS Level II Coding

Modifiers are an essential component of the HCPCS Level II coding system, just as they are of the CPT coding system. Modifiers convey extra information about the service or object, such as whether it is new or used, whether it is rented or purchased, etc. Modifiers may be found in phrases like "new and used," "rented and purchased," and so on. For instance, in our earlier illustration, if the oxygen equipment was rented, the provider would attach the modifier "RR" (Rental) to the code, so changing it to E0424RR to reflect the fact that the equipment was rented.

Helpful Hints for Accurately Coding HCPCS Level II

Here are a few pointers to assure correctness for individuals who are unfamiliar with this coding system:

1. Acquire an Awareness of the Coding Requirements: The Centers for Medicare & Medicaid Services (CMS) provide comprehensive instructions for utilizing HCPCS Level II codes. It is essential that you get yourself acquainted with these.

2. Make sure you are using the appropriate year's code book: The HCPCS Level II codes are modernized on a yearly basis. Check to see that you are utilizing the codebook for the current year.

3. Remember to Keep an Eye on the Modifiers: As was mentioned before, the coding scheme in question requires the use of modifiers. Be sure that you understand them and that you use that understanding effectively.

4. "Requirements for the Payer of the Check:" There is a possibility that various insurance carriers will have varying restrictions for the utilization of HCPCS Level II codes. Always make sure you are familiar with the relevant payer's policy.

The Importance of HCPCS Level II Codes for the Practice of Telemedicine

HCPCS codes are finding more and more applications as a result of the proliferation of telemedicine, particularly in the aftermath of the COVID-19 epidemic. HCPCS codes are assigned to a wide variety of the services that can be delivered through telemedicine, including remote patient monitoring and virtual check-ins. These services have provided healthcare practitioners with a whole new channel via which they may continue to give treatment to patients, even in situations where it is not possible for them to see patients in person. It is becoming increasingly vital for coders to demonstrate a mastery of understanding the right usage of HCPCS codes in this setting.

The HCPCS Level II Codes are a vital tool for coders to have at their disposal in the intricate industry that is medical billing and coding. They offer a standardized manner of reporting services and materials, which ensures that healthcare practitioners will be accurately reimbursed for their work. A comprehensive comprehension of these codes is an essential stepping stone on the path to becoming an expert in medical coding, which you are just starting out on. Take your time, put in some practice, and before you know it, you'll be able to deftly navigate this essential component of the world of code.

Essentials of ICD-10-CM Diagnosis Coding

When one enters the realm of medical coding, they will undoubtedly come across the International Classification of Diseases, Tenth Revision, Clinical Modification, more often known as ICD-10-CM. This system was developed by the World Health Organization (WHO), and the Centers for Disease Control and Prevention (CDC) and the National Center for Health Statistics (NCHS) modified it for use in the United States. It is an essential tool for classifying and coding all diagnoses, as well as certain procedures, for healthcare encounters.

Getting to Grips with ICD-10-CM Diagnosis Codes

ICD-10-CM codes are utilized in order to accurately depict the state of a patient. They record information on illnesses, signs, symptoms, aberrant findings, and the environmental factors that contribute to disease. These numbers are essential for billing purposes, as well as for reporting quality, compiling population health data, and monitoring diseases.

ICD-10-CM codes are completely unique and can include anything from three to seven characters each. The initial character is usually a letter, and it denotes a specific subset of illnesses or health problems. The second and third letters are also numeric, and they identify the particular region or etiology that is related with the sickness or health condition. Characters four through seven are a collection of letters and numbers that offer further information about the sickness or condition, such as the severity, laterality, and episode of treatment. These characters are found after the first three characters in the code.

Application of ICD-10-CM Codes in Real-World Settings

Take, for instance, the case of a patient who has been identified as having type 2 diabetes and moderate, no proliferative diabetic retinopathy with macular edema as their primary diagnosis. The comparable code in ICD-10-CM is E11.321, which can be found here.

The letter "E" in the first place of the code indicates that it pertains to conditions that are related to the endocrine system, nutrition, and metabolism.
The number "11" that comes after it clarifies that the disease in question is diabetes type 2.
Additional information on the nature and extent of the complication is provided by the ".321" extension.

The Importance of Being Specific When Coding with the ICD-10-CM

Because they are so thorough, ICD-10-CM codes make it possible to accurately code the ailments of patients. This level of detail is significant for a few reasons, including the following:

1. Better tracking of patients' ailments and how they are responding to therapy over time is made possible by detailed diagnostic codes, which contribute to improved patient care.

2. Accurate compensation: The more exact the diagnostic code is, the more correctly it represents the resources that were utilized in the patient's treatment, which ultimately leads to proper compensation.
3. The data on public health include detailed codes that assist in the identification of public health trends, the tracking of the spread of disease, and the informing of choices on health policy.

Coding Advice for Accurate Use of the ICD-10-CM
Due to the vast number of codes and the amount of specificity that is necessary, mastering ICD-10-CM coding might appear to be an insurmountable task. Nevertheless, if you follow these guidelines, you should find the procedure to be more manageable:

1. Acquire a Comprehensive Understanding of the Guidelines: The ICD-10-CM Official Guidelines for Coding and Reporting provide information that is crucial for learning how to utilize the ICD-10-CM coding system in the correct manner.
2. Remain Current: Because coding systems are changed on a regular basis, it is essential to remain current with the many modifications and upgrades that occur. utilize the Most Recent Version of the ICD-10-CM Coding handbook Always utilize the most recent version of the ICD-10-CM coding handbook to verify that you are utilizing legitimate, up-to-date codes.
4. Practice, Practice, and More Practice: Just like with any other ability, the more you practice coding, the better you'll get at it.

The Importance of Coding According to ICD-10-CM in Risk Adjustment

The function of ICD-10-CM coding in risk adjustment is the final factor to take into consideration. Risk adjustment models are utilized in the process of forecasting the expenses associated with medical treatment on the basis of diseases and demographic characteristics. Coding that is accurate and detailed according to the ICD-10-CM is essential for the successful operation of these models. Incomplete or inaccurate coding can result in a patient's health risk being incorrectly estimated and, as a consequence, in inadequate reimbursement for their medical treatment.

As a result, the ICD-10-CM diagnostic coding system serves as the foundation for medical billing and coding, having an impact on patient care as well as healthcare policy and reimbursement. To effectively navigate this system, you will need to have a solid grasp of its complexities and maintain a level of awareness regarding the many updates it undergoes. You may become an expert in this critical facet of medical coding with enough practice and determination, so improving the precision of health data collecting and making a contribution to the process of providing healthcare in its entirety.

Book 4: Reimbursement, Compliance, and Best Practices

Medical Billing and Reimbursement Processes

A medical bill goes through a maze-like process from the moment a patient schedules an appointment until the payment is collected and recorded, beginning with the patient making the appointment. It is a difficult procedure that calls for accuracy, careful attention to detail, and a profound familiarity with healthcare codes, insurance policies, and federal and state rules. Accurate compensation for services performed may be ensured by having a thorough understanding of this procedure, which can lead to increased financial security for healthcare practitioners.

The Continuum of a Medical Bill's Existence

In most cases, the following steps are required to complete the billing and reimbursement process for medical services:

1. Registration of Patients: The first step is when the patient calls to schedule an appointment. During registration, the demographic information and insurance information of the patient are gathered.

2. "Verification of Your Insurance:" The healthcare practitioner will verify the patient's insurance coverage in order to ascertain which services are covered by the patient's plan and how much the patient will be responsible for paying out of pocket.

3. "Check-In" and "Check-Out" Procedures for Patients: During these stages, the client's motive for visiting is determined, and the necessary services are offered. It is the patient's duty to pay any out-of-pocket expenses, such as copayments or deductibles, which are collected.

4. Coding in the Medical Field: By utilizing classification schemes like as ICD-10-CM, HCPCS Level II, and CPT, the diagnoses and operations that are carried out may be converted into standardized codes.

5. Entry on the Charge: The appropriate costs for the coded services are determined based on the fee schedule maintained by the healthcare provider.

6. Submission of the Claim The medical claim, which contains all of the coded services and expenses, is submitted to the insurance company in order to be reimbursed.

7. "Payment Posting": This refers to the process in which payments that have been received from both the patient and the insurance company are entered in the patient's account.

8. Follow-up and Appeals: In the event that a claim is rejected entirely or only partially paid for, the medical biller will research the cause for the rejection, make any necessary corrections, and then either resubmit the claim or file an appeal.

Comprehending the Terms of Payer Contracts

It is essential for healthcare providers to have a thorough understanding of the terms of the contracts they have with insurance payers in order to obtain correct compensation. The reimbursement rates for services, billing rules, and deadlines for claim submission are all outlined in these contracts. Claims that are denied or underpaid can be avoided by checking these contracts on a regular basis and keeping up with any modifications that may occur.

The Function of Electronic Health Records (EHRs) in the Healthcare System

In the process of paying and being reimbursed for services, Electronic Health Records (EHRs) are extremely important. They are responsible for the storage of patient data, the recording of services rendered, and frequently make first coding suggestions. Electronic health records have the potential to simplify and speed up the billing process, as well as minimize the number of mistakes that occur.

Helpful Hints for Accurately Billing Medical Services

The following are some helpful hints and guidelines for accurate and timely medical billing:

1. Always Check the Patient's Insurance Coverage Before delivering Services Always check the patient's insurance coverage before delivering services in order to avoid payment complications in the future.

2. "Code Accurately": Make certain that the coding correctly reflects the services that were rendered. Claim denials are possible outcomes of incorrect coding.

3. Quickly Submit Your Claims: The faster a claim is processed, the faster it will be paid. A timely filing helps avoid having a claim denied because it was submitted too late.

4. Continuously Follow Up: Continuously follow up on claims that have not been paid. When a claim is left unpaid for an extended period of time, it can become increasingly difficult to collect the money that is owed.

The Value-Based Reimbursement Model Is the Way of the Future in Medical Billing

As we look to the future, one of the most major changes that will take place in the healthcare system is the transition from fee-for-service to value-based compensation. Instead of being rewarded for the amount of services they give, healthcare practitioners under this model are rewarded for the quality of care they deliver. For the purpose of demonstrating beneficial results for patients, the gathering and reporting of accurate data is essential in this paradigm. It will be very necessary, in order to achieve success in the future healthcare landscape, to have an understanding of this altering paradigm and to change billing procedures accordingly.

The process of medical billing and reimbursement is a complex dance that demands careful attention to detail, careful attention to detail, thoroughness, and patience. You can safeguard the financial health of your practice and contribute to the general running of the healthcare system by having an awareness of this process, keeping up with changes, and adjusting to new reimbursement models.

Coding Compliance and Auditing

Coding compliance and auditing is a process that ensures accuracy, consistency, and adherence to coding standards and regulations; it is an essential aspect of healthcare administration. This area of healthcare not only ensures accurate accounting and reimbursement, but also aids in maintaining data integrity, which is essential for health information management, quality care, and informed decision-making.

The Importance of Compliance Coding

Coding compliance is the observance of coding guidelines and conventions established by organizations such as the American Medical Association (AMA) and the World Health Organization (WHO). It also entails adhering to federal and state regulations regarding the invoicing and coding of healthcare services.

A comprehensive coding compliance program is indispensable to an organization for multiple reasons:

1. Accurate Reimbursement: Adherence to correct classification practices assures an accurate reflection of the medical services rendered, thereby resulting in accurate reimbursement.

2. Avoiding Legal Consequences: Noncompliance can lead to examinations by regulatory bodies, legal penalties, and sanctions.

3. Quality Patient Care: Correct coding results in accurate patient data, which is essential for quality care, research, and health policy decisions.

Auditing's Importance for Coding Compliance

Auditing is the process of systematically scrutinizing coding and billing practices to identify errors, inconsistencies, and deviations from standard coding practices. Routine audits can aid in:

1. Identify Coding Errors: Audits can uncover coding errors such as incorrect code assignment, under coding or over coding, and unbundling of codes.
Regular audits can assist an organization in remaining compliant with ever-changing healthcare regulations, thereby reducing the possibility of incurring fines.

2. Improve Revenue Cycle Management: By identifying and correcting coding errors, audits can result in accurate reimbursement and enhanced revenue cycle management.

Implementing a Program for Coding Compliance and Auditing

Listed below are some stages for establishing an effective compliance and auditing program for coding:

1. Develop a Compliance Plan: It is essential to have a well-defined, documented compliance plan. It should delineate the organization's commitment to compliance, define coding standards, describe the audit procedure, and detail the repercussions of noncompliance.
2. Regular Training and Education: Regular training and education for coding employees on coding standards, revisions, and best practices is essential for maintaining compliance.
3. Conduct Regular Audits: Regular internal and external audits can help identify and correct issues before they escalate.
4. Corrective Action: Take prompt corrective action if an audit reveals issues. This could involve retraining, process enhancement, or disciplinary action in some instances.

Risk Adjustment and HCC Coding: The Future of Compliance Coding and Auditing

In the foreseeable future, risk adjustment and Hierarchical Condition Category (HCC) coding will become increasingly crucial. Chronic conditions are represented by HCC codes in risk adjustment models, which are used to predict healthcare costs based on conditions and demographic factors.

Correct risk adjustment necessitates accurate HCC categorization. As we move toward a value-based healthcare model, understanding risk adjustment and HCC coding will be essential for coding compliance. Regular audits can ensure accuracy in these areas, leading to a correct representation of patient complexity and an accurate estimation of healthcare costs.

Essentially, coding compliance and auditing are not only about following rules and avoiding penalties. They are concerned with maintaining the accuracy and integrity of health information, enhancing patient care, and ensuring the financial stability of healthcare organizations. You can confidently navigate the coding maze and contribute to the overall efficacy of your organization by implementing a robust compliance program and conducting regular audits.

CPC Exam Tips and Best Practices

On the path to becoming a professional medical coder, the Certified Professional Coder (CPC) exam is a major milestone. A thorough understanding of medical coding procedures, anatomy, and medical terminology is required to pass this exam. Nevertheless, with adequate planning and strategies, you can overcome this obstacle.

Understanding the CPC Examination Format

The American Academy of Professional Coders (AAPC) administers the CPC exam, which consists of 150 multiple-choice questions that must be answered within 5 hours and 40 minutes. The examination covers numerous subjects, including:

1. Medical Coding: This includes knowledge of ICD-10-CM, CPT, and HCPCS Level II coding.
2. Anatomy and Physiology: You must comprehend the systems of the human body and how they operate.
3. Medical Terminology: The examination assesses your knowledge of the terminology used to describe symptoms, conditions, treatments, and procedures.
4. Compliance and Regulatory: You must be conversant with medical coding-related laws and regulations.

Effective Study Techniques

Given the scope and profundity of the CPC exam, an effective study plan is required. Here are some techniques:

1. Build a Study Schedule: Allocate regular, consistent study times in your schedule. Vary the subjects that you study during each study session to make them more manageable.
2. Comprehension of Coding Guidelines: Comprehension of the coding conventions and guidelines for ICD-10-CM, CPT, and HCPCS Level II.

3. Practice with Real Scenarios: To reinforce your comprehension, practice coding with actual medical records.

4. Take Sample Tests: The AAPC provides practice exams that mimic the actual exam. These can assist you in familiarizing yourself with the format of the exam and identifying areas in which you need to improve.

Guidelines for Exam Day

On the day of the exam, consider the following suggestions for optimal performance:

1. Manage Your Time: With less than two minutes per question, time management is critical. Skip difficult questions and come back to them if you have time left.

2. Use Your Books: The exam is open book, so make sure your coding manuals are well-organized and tabbed for quick reference.

3. Carefully Read the Questions: Misreading a query can result in an incorrect response. Take your time to comprehend the question's intent.

4. Remain Calm and Concentrated: It is normal to feel anxious, but strive to remain composed. Deep breathing exercises can aid in relaxation and concentration.

Maintenance of Your CPC Certification

Remember that your learning voyage will continue even after you have passed the CPC exam. Every two years, you must complete 36 continuing education units (CEUs) to maintain your CPC certification. These can be obtained through webinars, conferences, online courses, and other means.

Medical coding is beginning to be affected by advancements in healthcare technology. For example, the use of electronic health records (EHRs) is growing in popularity. As you advance in your medical coding career, seek out opportunities to familiarize yourself with EHRs, as such knowledge can make you a more effective and in-demand professional.

The CPC examination may appear intimidating, but you can approach it with confidence if you have the proper preparation and strategies. Remember that the path to becoming a certified professional coder entails not only completing an exam, but also embracing a career of lifelong learning and adaptation to the ever-changing healthcare environment.

Book 5: Comprehensive CPC Exam Preparation

Medical Terminology Review

It is absolutely necessary for anyone working in the healthcare profession to have a thorough grasp of medical terminology. It is the global language that helps professionals from different fields, like as physicians, nurses, coders, and billers, communicate more effectively with one another and bridges any gaps that may exist between them. It is not only a matter of vocabulary for those who work in the medical field; rather, it is essential to accurate diagnosis, treatment, and billing.

The Building Blocks of Medical Terminology

When broken down into its component parts, medical terminology consists of a variety of components that, if comprehended, may assist in the interpretation of even the most convoluted jargon. These components include the following:

1. Root Words: These are the fundamental parts of a term that most frequently designate a system or a component of the body. For instance, the name "cardiology" derives from the prefix "cardio-," which is a reference to the heart.
2. [Prefixes:] [Prefixes:] In order to change the meaning of root words, they are appended to the beginning of the terms. For example, the word "hypoglycemia" begins with the prefix "hypo-," which means "low" or "under," and refers to an abnormally low level of glucose in the blood.
3. "Suffixes" are added to the end of root words to signify a condition, disease, or treatment. Suffixes can also stand alone as standalone nouns. In the medical term 'otitis,' the suffix 'itis' indicates inflammation, while the prefix 'oto-' refers to the ear.

Methods for Achieving Proficient Knowledge of Medical Terminology

Given the sheer amount of phrases involved, it's easy to feel overwhelmed while trying to learn medical vocabulary. Nevertheless, if one employs the appropriate tactics, one can successfully complete the work at hand:

1. Determine the Root, Prefix, and Suffix of a Word First, it is important to determine the root, prefix, and suffix of a word before attempting to comprehend more complicated medical terminology. In this method, you will be able to comprehend the meaning of the phrase by referring to the meanings of its constituent parts.

2. Make use of flashcards by writing the phrase on one side of the card and the definition on the other side of the flashcard. Reviewing these flashcards on a consistent basis might assist to strengthen your memory.

3. Commit to a Regular Practice: Committing to a Regular Practice is Essential. In order to get more familiar with the phrases, include medical language into your day-to-day activities.

The Importance of Terminology in the Field of Medicine and Healthcare

It is essential to have a solid grasp of medical terminology in many different areas of healthcare, including the following:

1. In clinical practice, it is imperative that healthcare professionals effectively communicate a patient's symptoms, diagnosis, and treatment options in order to ensure the patient's safety.

2. "Medical Coding and Billing": A comprehensive knowledge of medical terminology is required for the accurate translation of medical records into coded form for the purposes of billing.

3. Healthcare Administration: Knowledge of medical language can be helpful for administrators in comprehending medical reports, keeping health records, and making choices that are based on accurate information.

A Look Back at the Development of Medical Terminology

The vocabulary used in medicine is always evolving. It develops in tandem with advances in medical research and technology. The discovery of novel diseases, therapies, and technology frequently results in the coining of new names. For example, words like "telemedicine" and "personalized medicine" have evolved as a result of developments in both technological capabilities and therapeutic strategies.

As a healthcare provider, it is essential for you to keep up with the latest medical terminology and thinking. You may assist yourself keep up with the rapidly changing environment of medical terminology by participating in regular training, continuing your education, and keeping up with the latest medical breakthroughs.

Although difficult to understand, medical language is an essential component of effective healthcare communication. You may acquire a solid foundation in this global language by first gaining a knowledge of its structure, and then consistently practicing the usage of that framework. It is important to keep in mind that acquiring knowledge of medical terminology is not simply about memorization of phrases; rather, it is about improving communication, protecting the safety of patients, and contributing to the provision of quality healthcare.

Anatomy Review

The human body, which is an amazing collection of many systems that are all related to one another, is the foundation of health and medicine. The study of anatomy, which focuses on the structure of the human body, is essential for anyone working in the medical field. This knowledge is helpful in the diagnosis of illnesses, the formulation of treatment strategies, and the performance of medical operations.

Essential Components of the Human Body

Gross (Macroscopic) Anatomy and Microscopic Anatomy are the two primary divisions that are often utilized in the study of human anatomy.

1. Gross Anatomy: This is the study of the parts of the body that can be observed with the naked eye. It may then be further broken down into:

- Regional Anatomy is the study of all of the structures that are located in a certain region of the body.
   Systematic anatomy is the study of the human body in terms of its many systems, including the circulatory system, the neurological system, and so on.

2. The study of microscopic anatomy: This subfield examines phenomena that require the use of a microscope to be observed by the naked eye alone, as the name indicates. It includes the following:

- Histology may be defined as the study of tissues.

- The study of cells is referred to as cytology.

Developing Your Understanding of the Anatomy

Due to the vast amount of material available, studying anatomy might feel like an uphill battle at times. Nevertheless, if one employs the appropriate tactics, one may successfully deal with it:

1. Get a grasp on the big picture: To begin, you need to have an awareness of how the many physiological systems interact with one another. This will give a framework for understanding the many components that make up the whole.
2. Make Use of Visual Aids: Diagrams, models, and movies may be quite helpful when attempting to visualize the spatial relationships between different structures.
3. Engage in consistent practice: Regular study and testing of one's own knowledge can assist to strengthen one's memory.

The Role of Anatomy in Medical Care

The following are some of the ways in which anatomy is essential to the practice of medicine:

1. "Patient Assessment": In this step of the healthcare process, clinicians utilize their knowledge of anatomy to evaluate patients, get an understanding of the symptoms they are experiencing, and select a treatment plan.
2. Medical operations: Whether it's surgery or just a simple injection, all medical operations require an in-depth knowledge of anatomy. This is true regardless of the type of technique being performed.
3. Medical Imaging: In order to interpret X-rays, MRIs, and other imaging, you need to have knowledge of normal anatomy in addition to its deviations.

The Evolving Characteristics of the Anatomical Structure

Although the fundamental make-up of the human body does not change, our knowledge of it constantly expands even as it stays the same. The findings of recent study frequently shed light on previously unknown parts of anatomy. For example, recent developments have led to a greater knowledge of the microanatomy of the brain as well as the intricate interaction of neurons.

Furthermore, when medical technology progresses, we frequently find that our understanding of anatomy has to be reexamined in light of these advancements. Educating students about anatomy today makes use of cutting-edge technologies like virtual and augmented reality, which provide experiences that are both immersive and engaging.

System of the Skeletons

The skeletal system in our bodies serves as the primary support structure for our bodies, as well as providing protection for the internal organs, assisting in mobility, and performing a number of other important roles. When learning about the human skeleton, it's best to start with broad categories like the axial and appendicular skeletons, and then work your way down to the individual bones. Remember that it's not only about learning the names of the bones; it's also about understanding the distinctive characteristics of each bone and the tasks they serve.

The System of the Muscles

Movement, stability, and the creation of heat are all tasks that are completed by the muscular system. First, familiarize yourself with the major muscle groups, and then work your way down to the individual muscles. Acquire a working knowledge of the origin, insertion, action, and innervation of each muscle. When trying to comprehend the musculoskeletal system, visual aids can be of tremendous assistance.

System of the Cardiovascular

The cardiovascular system, which consists of the heart and the veins that carry blood throughout the body, is in charge of supplying oxygen and nutrients to all parts of the body as well as being responsible for the circulation of blood. First, you should become familiar with the anatomy of the heart and the course that blood takes through the body before moving on to the vascular system. To have a complete understanding of the cardiovascular system, it is necessary to be familiar with both its anatomy and its physiology.

System of the Nerves

The nervous system serves as the body's command and control center. The brain and spinal cord make up the central nervous system, whereas nerves throughout the body make up the peripheral nervous system. Because of the intricate nature of the neural system, a methodical approach is very necessary. You should begin with the overall organization, and then go on to focusing on particular areas or components.

The Breathing and Breathing System

The respiratory system, which is made up of the organs that are in charge of breathing, is an essential component in the process of gas exchange. Study the mechanics of breathing after first learning about the upper respiratory system, then moving on to the lower respiratory tract, and lastly beginning with the upper respiratory tract.

System of Digestive Organs

The digestive system is responsible for breaking down food, removing nutrients, and eliminating waste. Beginning in the mouth cavity, trace the way that food travels through the various organs of the body.

Keep in mind that learning anatomy takes time and effort. This is not a race; rather, it is a marathon. Make learning an active process rather than a passive one. Make diagrams, participate in collaborative research, share what you've learned with others, and put your skills to use in real-world scenarios whenever you can. Maintain an awareness of the most recent findings from research and improvements in medical technology, and never stop looking for new ways to improve your comprehension and memory.

Last but not least, make sure you never lose sight of the fact that the ultimate purpose of studying anatomy is to be able to use what you've learned to better the treatment that patients get. Always ask yourself, when you gain a new understanding of a topic, "How does this concept relate to the health of the patient?" What specific ways can I expect this to improve my performance as a healthcare professional? If you keep these questions in mind when you're studying anatomy, you'll discover that it's not only rewarding but also important to your future profession. Keep in mind that mastering anatomy takes time and constant effort over many years. It is not enough to just commit the names and locations of various bodily parts to memory; one must also comprehend how these components interact with one another in order to sustain life. Therefore, go out on this adventure with an open mind and plenty of perseverance. As you learn more, you'll develop an appreciation for the intricate beauty that is the human body and the intricate beauty that is its functioning. Your newfound understanding of anatomy will prove to be a very useful asset throughout your career in the medical field. It will enable you to comprehend the complexities of the human body and make a more significant contribution to the improvement of patient care.

Full-length Test 1

Medical Terminology and Anatomy

1. Which of the following prefixes means "around"?
a) endo-
b) circum-
c) meta-
d) hyper-

2. The study of tissues is called:
a) Cytology
b) Histology
c) Physiology
d) Pathology

3. Which bodily process involves eosinophils?
a) Blood clotting
b) Inflammation
c) Temperature regulation
d) Chemical digestion

4. Which abdominal organ produces bile?
a) Pancreas
b) Liver
c) Gallbladder
d) Small intestine

5. The myocardium comprises which of the following tissue layers of the heart?
a) Epicardium
b) Endocardium
c) Pericardium
d) Myocardium

6. What is the anatomical term for the back of the knee?
a) Patella
b) Popliteal fossa
c) Olecranon
d) Calcaneus

7. Which medical abbreviation indicates "before meals"?
a) bid
b) hs
c) ac
d) pc

ICD-10-CM Coding Guidelines

8. What is the sequencing priority for encounters for rehabilitation services?
a) The condition requiring rehabilitation
b) The reason for the encounter
c) Any associated complications
d) No sequencing guidelines apply

9. Which of the following conditions is classified as an acute form versus a chronic form in ICD-10-CM?
a) Diabetes
b) Asthma
c) Liver disease
d) Hypertension

10. When assigning a diagnosis code, a coder should:
a) Code only confirmed diagnoses
b) Query the provider for clarification
c) Select the code for highest degree of specificity
d) Assign codes for all documented conditions

11. What is the appropriate code assignment for a patient with type 2 diabetes mellitus and diabetic peripheral angiopathy?
a) E08.51, E11.51
b) E11.9, E08.51
c) E11.9
d) E08.51

12. Which guideline states that codes ending in "A" should not be used for HIPAA reporting?
a) Signs & Symptoms
b) Injuries
c) Use of External Cause Codes
d) Level of Detail

13. How should multiple lumpectomy procedures be coded?
a) Code to the number of lumpectomy procedures performed
b) Code multiple lumpectomies as a single procedure

c) Assign left and right-side codes
d) Assign codes for lumpectomy and re-excision

14. What is the timeframe for coding recent versus chronic conditions?
a) Less than 8 weeks
b) 4-6 weeks
c) Less than 3 months
d) It is not defined

ICD-10-CM Coding

15. Which ICD-10-CM code identifies a pressure ulcer of the right lower back?
a) L89.153
b) L89.154
c) L89.156
d) L89.159

16. A patient is admitted for observation following a motor vehicle accident. Which diagnosis code should be reported as principal for the admission?
a) Z04.1
b) Z04.3
c) Z04.4
d) Z04.9

17. A patient presents with right knee pain and a suspected old bucket handle tear of the medial meniscus.

Which ICD-10-CM code is correct?
a) M25.562
b) M23.50x
c) M23.502
d) M23.6x2

18. Which code identifies acute viral pharyngitis?
a) J00
b) J02.0
c) J02.9
d) J06.9

19. Which malignancy of bronchus code indicates the left side?
a) C34.31
b) C34.32
c) C34.311
d) C34.312

20. A patient is treated for systolic heart failure. What code should be assigned?
a) I50.1
b) I50.20
c) I50.30
d) I50.9

21. Which code indicates a displaced left hip fracture?
a) S72.001B
b) S72.002B
c) S72.009A
d) S72.019B

CPT Coding Guidelines

22. What is the appropriate way to code for a procedure performed on multiple structures in the same organ?
a) Code to each procedure separately
b) Code only the most extensive procedure
c) Code multiple procedures with modifier 51
d) Code based on surgical approach

23. Which of the following factors determine the order in which codes should be sequenced?
a) The reason for the encounter
b) Degree of complexity
c) AHIMA guidelines
d) Payor guidelines

24. According to CPT guidelines, you may need to assign separate codes for different anatomic sites during the same encounter if the sites are ___.
a) Contiguous
b) Non-contiguous
c) Bilateral
d) Ipsilateral

25. What is the definition of an add-on code in the CPT Manual?
a) Additional procedure at another encounter

b) Procedure not normally reported alone
c) Related evaluation and management service
d) Secondary procedure performed with highest RVU

26. Category III codes are:
a) Temporary codes for emerging technology
b) Permanent codes for routine services
c) Required for correct coding
d) Used to bypass NCCI edits

27. Which modifier would be appropriate for coding a procedure performed on the left side?
a) 50
b) LC
c) LT
d) -59

28. Unspecified CPT codes should be used:
a) When a more specific code exists
b) Only if directed by a payor policy
c) As a last option only
d) For unlisted services only

CPT Coding
29. What is the appropriate CPT code for a colonoscopy with snare removal of a colon polyp?
a) 45380
b) 45385
c) 45384
d) 45388

30. Which CPT code represents a coronary artery bypass graft of a single vessel?
a) 33510
b) 33511
c) 33512
d) 33513

31. A patient undergoes incision of an ischiorectal abscess. What is the correct code?
a) 46040
b) 46050
c) 46060
d) 46221

32. What CPT code is reported for a vaginal hysterectomy that includes removal of tubes and ovaries?
a) 58150
b) 58553
c) 58554
d) 58541

33. Which CPT code represents a low complexity established patient office visit?
a) 99211
b) 99212
c) 99213
d) 99214

34. What is the appropriate coding for closed treatment of a nondisplaced ankle fracture?
a) 27750
b) 27814
c) 27816
d) 27822

35. Which modifier indicates a procedure was discontinued?
a) 73
b) 52
c) 53
d) 74

HCPCS Coding
36. What type of items are assigned codes in the HCPCS Level II system?
a) Procedures
b) Services
c) Supplies
d) Drugs

37. Which section of HCPCS codes represents temporary national codes?
a) A codes
b) B codes
c) C codes
d) Q codes

38. To bill for injectable drugs, a provider must report the CPT injection code and the appropriate HCPCS code for the:

a) Drug amount
b) Injection site
c) Drug type
d) Number of units administered

39. Which modifier is used with HCPCS Level II DME codes?
a) RR
b) NU
c) UE
d) RA

40. What HCPCS code represents a manual wheelchair?
a) K0001
b) K0005
c) K0009
d) E1161

41. Billing for discarded drug amounts uses which HCPCS modifier?
a) JA
b) JW
c) 59
d) 25

42. According to guidelines, HCPCS codes may be reported in addition to the _____ code.
a) ASA
b) ASP
c) APC
d) CPT

Modifiers
43. Which modifier is used to indicate a procedure was performed on the left upper eyelid?
a) E3
b) FA
c) LT
d) LU

44. When is it appropriate to use modifier 59?
a) To indicate distinct procedural services
b) When a procedure is partially reduced
c) To bypass an NCCI edit
d) For bilateral procedures

45. Which modifier indicates an assistant surgeon?
a) AS
b) 80
c) 81
d) 82

46. What modifier is reported with the administration CPT code for a discarded drug amount?
a) JA
b) JB
c) JW\
d) JO

47. Modifier -25 should be appended to an E/M service on the same date as a procedure when the:
a) Decision to perform surgery is made

b) Visit warrants a separately identifiable E/M service
c) Patient is scheduled for a return procedure
d) Preoperative workup is documented

48. The physician modifier -57 is used to indicate:
a) Bilateral procedures
b) Distinct procedural services
c) Reduced services
d) Decision for surgery

49. Which modifier would indicate continued therapy services?
a) 76
b) 77
c) 78
d) 79

Anesthesia Coding
50. To calculate anesthesia time, the anesthesia start time is documented when the anesthesiologist begins to:
a) Administer anesthesia
b) Prepare the patient
c) Review the medical record
d) Monitor the patient

51. When coding anesthesia, the base value assigned

represents anesthesia services for the first ____ of time.
a) 15 minutes
b) 30 minutes
c) 45 minutes
d) 60 minutes

52. Which of the following does NOT impact anesthesia code selection?
a) Duration
b) Physical status
c) Surgical procedure
d) Age of the patient

53. When a patient stop breathing during general anesthesia, what code is reported in addition to the regular anesthesia code?
a) 99100
b) 99116
c) 99135
d) 99140

54. Anesthesia time ends when the anesthesiologist is no longer in personal attendance with the patient.
a) True
b) False

55. Which physical status modifier indicates an emergency surgery?
a) P3
b) P4
c) P5

d) P6

56. What basic anesthesia code is reported for the first 30 minutes for a patient age 3?
a) 00140
b) 00150
c) 00160
d) 00170

E/M Coding

57. A detailed interval history, problem-focused ROS, and detailed exam are documented for an established patient office visit. What level of E/M service is supported?
a) 99211
b) 99212
c) 99213
d) 99214

58. What constitutes the chief complaint in E/M services?
a) CC
b) HPI
c) ROS
d) PFSH

59. To meet criteria for a detailed history, documentation must include ___ elements from the HPI.
a) 1-3
b) 4+
c) 6-8
d) 10+

60. Physical exam levels for office/outpatient services are based on ___ of systems examined.
a) Number
b) Extent
c) Complexity
d) Severity

61. Billing both an inpatient hospital visit and an office visit on the same day by the same physician requires what modifier?
a) 24
b) 25
c) 27
d) 57

62. Which types of documentation may be used to support an E/M service level?
a) ROS & Exam only
b) HPI & MDM only
c) HPI, Exam, MDM
d) Any 2 of 3 key components

63. What E/M code represents a moderate complexity established patient office visit?
a) 99212
b) 99213
c) 99214
d) 99215

Radiology Coding

64. To code contrast used during an MRI procedure, the coder must know the _____.
a) Volume administered
b) Injection site
c) Type of equipment used
d) Radiologist's credentials

65. What is the difference between codes for MRI of the right knee with and without contrast?
a) G codes
b) Anatomic specificity
c) Time of service
d) Radiologist qualifications

66. Which modifier indicates that the radiology service is for diagnostic versus screening purposes?
a) CT
b) LC
c) LD
d) RT

67. When a radiologic exam is terminated due to an allergy to contrast, which modifier should be appended?
a) -52
b) -73
c) -74
d) -LT

68. Which of the following does NOT affect code selection for diagnostic imaging services?
a) Body region imaged
b) Whether contrast was used
c) Radiologist interpretation
d) Who performed the service

69. To code for fluoroscopy guidance, the time should be documented in ____.
a) 15 minute increments
b) Minutes
c) Hours
d) No time is needed

70. An x-ray of the right foot is taken with three views. What is the correct coding?
a) 73610
b) 73610 x 3
c) 73615
d) 73615 x 3

Pathology and Laboratory Coding

71. A biopsy of breast tissue is performed. Which code represents the pathology for interpretation and report?
a) 88104
b) 88305
c) 88307

d) 88309

72. When coding Pap smears, the type of cervical source is represented by the:
a) First digit
b) Second digit
c) Third digit
d) Fifth digit

73. To code for a urinalysis, the coder must know documentation of the:
a) Urine appearance
b) Number examined
c) Method performed
d) Corpuscle count

74. What CPT code represents a basic metabolic panel?
a) 80047
b) 80048
c) 80050
d) 80053

75. Modifier 90 would be appended to the HCPCS code for:
a) Serum sodium level
b) Fasting glucose
c) Bleeding time test
d) Therapeutic drug monitoring

76. Which lab test assesses cardiac enzyme levels?
a) 82009
b) 82017
c) 82042
d) 83026

77. To report a surgical pathology gross and microscopic exam, which modifier is used?
a) 26
b) 47
c) 59
d) 91

Medicine Coding

78. A patient presents with a cough, fever, and green sputum production. Which ICD-10 code represents acute bronchitis?
a) J40
b) J41.0
c) J42
d) J44.9

79. What ICD-10 code is assigned for a patient with Type 2 diabetes mellitus with diabetic nephropathy?
a) E08.21
b) E09.21
c) E10.21
d) E11.21

80. A patient is treated for a stage III pressure ulcer on the right hip. What is the correct ICD-10 code?
a) L89.13
b) L89.23
c) L89.33
d) L89.43

81. An adult patient undergoes tonsillectomy due to chronic tonsillitis. Which diagnosis code is reported as primary?
a) J03.90
b) J35.1
c) J35.3
d) R49.0

82. What ICD-10 code represents a displaced spiral fracture of the left femur?
a) S72.001B
b) S72.002B\
c) S72.009B
d) S72.091B

83. Type 2 diabetes mellitus with diabetic peripheral angiopathy is represented by which code?
a) E08.51
b) E09.51
c) E10.51
d) E11.51

84. Which code indicates a benign neoplasm of the thyroid?
a) C73
b) D09.3
c) D34
d) D44.9

Surgery Coding

85. What is the CPT code for a laparoscopic appendectomy?
a) 44950
b) 44960
c) 44970
d) 44799

86. Which CPT code represents the surgical extraction of four wisdom teeth?
a) D7111
b) D7210
c) D7220
d) D7230

87. What CPT code is reported for a vaginal hysterectomy with anterior and posterior colporrhaphy?
a) 58150
b) 58552
c) 58553
d) 58570

88. A right knee arthroscopy with meniscectomy is performed. What CPT code should be used?
a) 29870
b) 29873
c) 29874
d) 29877

89. What surgical approach is reported with CPT code 27130?
a) Open
b) Percutaneous
c) Arthroscopic
d) Percutaneous endoscopic

90. Which ICD-10 procedure code indicates an excisional breast biopsy?
a) 0HTU0ZZ
b) 0HTT0ZZ

c) 0HTV0ZZ
d) 0TBG0ZX

91. An adult patient undergoes a tonsillectomy due to chronic tonsillitis. What is the procedure code?
a) 42820
b) 42821
c) 42825
d) 42826

Inpatient Hospital Coding
92. What is the POA indicator used to identify diagnoses that develop after inpatient admission?
a) 0
b) 1
c) 2
d) 9

93. When assigning the principal diagnosis for inpatient coding, the coder should select the condition that:
a) Required the most resources
b) Prolonged the hospital stay
c) Was most severe
d) Caused admission

94. A patient is admitted for chest pain and has a family history of coronary artery disease. What is coded as principal diagnosis?

a) Family history
b) Chest pain
c) Suspected coronary artery disease
d) Likely angina pectoris

95. When a patient is readmitted within 30 days, which condition is sequenced first?
a) Original principal diagnosis
b) Reason for readmission
c) Unresolved complication
d) Any codeable condition

96. What is the ICD-10-PCS code for a PTCA of three coronary arteries with stents?
a) 02703DZ
b) 02703DZ, 02703DZ, 02703DZ
c) 02703D3
d) 02703D3, 02703D3, 02703D3

97. Splints and casting supplies are reported with which ICD-10-PCS section?
a) Medical and Surgical
b) Placement
c) Administration
d) Measurement and Monitoring

98. Mechanical ventilation for less than 96 hours is coded as:
a) 5A09357

b) 5A1935Z
c) 5A1945Z
d) 5A1955Z

HIPAA Compliance
99. Which of the following constitutes protected health information under HIPAA?
a) Patient name
b) Medical record number
c) Date of service
d) All of the above

100. HIPAA allows covered entities to use or disclose PHI without patient authorization for ___.
a) Treatment, payment, healthcare operations
b) Public health purposes
c) Reporting abuse, neglect or domestic violence
d) All of the above

101. Patients have the right to inspect and obtain a copy of their medical records under HIPAA.
a) True
b) False

102. The HIPAA Privacy Rule applies to which of the following?
a) Health plans

b) Healthcare providers
c) Healthcare clearinghouses
d) All of the above

103. Which HIPAA transaction standard facilitates electronic claims submission?
a) 270/271 - Eligibility inquiry and response
b) 276/277 - Claim status inquiry and response
c) 837 - Healthcare claim
d) 835 - Electronic remittance advice

104. HIPAA requires appropriate ___. to ensure the confidentiality and security of protected health information.
a) Physical safeguards
b) Administrative safeguards
c) Technical safeguards
d) All of the above

105. What is the penalty per HIPAA violation incident?
a) $50,000
b) $100,000
c) $250,000
d) $500,000

Reimbursement and Billing Procedures

106. An anesthesia record must document

the ___ to code for anesthesia services.
a) Type of anesthesia used
b) Procedure performed
c) Start and end times
d) ASA physical status

107. A re-submission of a previously denied claim is known as a/an ___.
a) Redetermination
b) Reconsideration
c) Appeal
d) Follow-up inquiry

108. Services provided as inpatient care must meet _____ criteria to receive reimbursement.
a) Medical necessity
b) Coding guidelines
c) Documentation standards
d) Bundling policies

109. What form is used by facilities to report outpatient services for reimbursement?
a) 1500 Health Insurance Claim Form
b) UB-04 Claim Form
c) CMS 1500
d) Outpatient Encounter Form

110. An EOB with the remark code "N385" indicates:
a) Timeframe for claim submission exceeded

b) Duplicate claim/service
c) Records indicate this patient has no coverage
d) Non-covered service

111. Under Medicare's fee-for-service, providers are reimbursed using which model?
a) Bundled payments
b) Capitation
c) Fee schedules
d) Value-based payments

112. Medical coding improves reimbursement through accurate representation of the _____ and resources required.
a) Payer contracts
b) Provider liability
c) Complexity of services\
d) Site of service

Ophthalmology and Otorhinolaryngology Coding

113. What is the CPT code for an intermediate office visit for an established patient with an ophthalmologist?
a) 92002
b) 92012
c) 92014

d) 92015

114. Which of the following procedures involves incision of tear ducts?
a) Dacryocystorhinostomy
b) Punctoplasty
c) Blepharoplasty
d) Keratoplasty

115. What CPT code represents a diagnostic nasal endoscopy?
a) 31237
b) 31500
c) 31575
d) 31579

116. Excision of a malignant lesion on the external ear is coded to biopsy code 11100 with the addition of what modifier?
a) 22
b) 25
c) 78
d) 90

117. Which ICD-10 code indicates acquired absence of the right eye?
a) Z90.01
b) H54.7
c) Q10.2
d) Q13.4

118. A stapedectomy is performed. What is the root operation?
a) Resection
b) Reposition

c) Alteration
d) Extraction

119. What procedure does CPT code 69436 represent?
a) Myringotomy
b) Mastoidectomy
c) Tympanostomy
d) Stapedectomy

Cardiovascular System Coding

120. What CPT code represents a right heart cardiac catheterization?
a) 93506
b) 93507
c) 93511
d) 93530

121. A patient undergoes an echocardiogram with Doppler for evaluation of suspected cardiomyopathy. What is the appropriate CPT code?
a) 93306
b) 93307
c) 93308
d) 93350

122. Which ICD-10-CM code indicates acute myocardial infarction of unspecified site?
a) I21.01
b) I21.9
c) I22.0
d) I25.2

123. What is the ICD-10-PCS code for a PTCA of a coronary artery using a drug-eluting stent?
a) 0270346
b) 02703DZ
c) 02703E3
d) 02703F3

124. A patient undergoes a CABG using a venous graft. What is the root operation?
a) Bypass
b) Transplantation
c) Resection
d) Fusion

125. Varicose veins of the right lower extremity with ulcer is coded as:
a) I83.811
b) I83.013
c) I83.813
d) I87.2

126. What procedure code describes surgical closure of a patent ductus arteriosus?
a) 33361
b) 33392
c) 33366
d) 33401

Gastroenterology Coding

127. What CPT code represents a diagnostic colonoscopy with biopsy?

a) 45378
b) 45380
c) 45383
d) 45385

128. A patient undergoes an EGD with biopsy. What CPT code is reported?
a) 43200
b) 43202
c) 43235
d) 43239

129. Which ICD-10-CM code indicates Crohn's disease of the small intestine?
a) K50.00
b) K50.012
c) K50.112
d) K50.812

130. What is the ICD-10-PCS code for a low anterior resection of the rectum?
a) 0DTN4ZZ
b) 0DTQ4ZZ
c) 0DTQ8ZZ
d) 0D5Q8ZZ

131. A feeding jejunostomy tube is placed. What is the approach?
a) Open
b) Percutaneous
c) Percutaneous Endoscopic
d) Via Natural or Artificial Opening

132. Endoscopic retrograde cholangiopancreatography (ERCP) maps to root operation:
a) Drainage
b) Extraction
c) Inspection
d) Reposition

133. What procedure does CPT code 47562 represent?
a) Diagnostic laparoscopy
b) Laparoscopic cholecystectomy
c) Laparoscopic appendectomy
d) Laparoscopic gastroenterostomy

Neurology and Psychiatry Coding

134. What CPT code represents a comprehensive neurological exam of a new patient?
a) 99201
b) 99202
c) 99205
d) 99281

135. Which ICD-10-CM code indicates classic migraine with intractable migraine with status migrainosus?
a) G43.001
b) G43.101
c) G43.111
d) G43.711

136. A spinal puncture is performed to obtain cerebrospinal fluid. What is the CPT code?
a) 62270
b) 62272
c) 62310
d) 62311

137. Partial motor epilepsy with impairment of consciousness is coded as:
a) G40.109
b) G40.111
c) G40.211
d) G40.219

138. A patient undergoes a cerebral angiogram. What is the root operation?
a) Restriction
b) Fluoroscopy
c) Inspection
d) Occlusion

139. What psychiatric disorder is characterized by irrational fears or phobias?
a) Bipolar disorder
b) Depression
c) Schizophrenia
d) Anxiety disorder

140. Which modality code represents electroconvulsive therapy?
a) GZB0ZZZ
b) GZB1ZZZ
c) GZB2ZZZ

d) GZB4ZZZ

Respiratory System Coding

141. What is the ICD-10-CM code for acute bronchitis due to respiratory syncytial virus?
a) J20.5
b) J20.8
c) J21.0
d) J21.9

142. A patient undergoes a diagnostic bronchoscopy. What is the CPT code?
a) 31622
b) 31625
c) 31628
d) 31629

143. Which ICD-10-PCS code indicates resection of apical lung bulla via thoracoscopic approach?
a) 0BB04ZX\
b) 0BBP4ZX
c) 0BBQ4ZX
d) 0BPQ4ZX

144. What CPT code represents intubation, endotracheal, emergency procedure?
a) 31500
b) 31502
c) 31500
d) 31505

145. ICD-10-CM code J44.9 represents diagnosis of:
a) Simple chronic bronchitis
b) Chronic asthmatic bronchitis
c) Chronic obstructive asthma
d) Unspecified chronic obstructive pulmonary disease

146. Which ICD-10-PCS approach is used for surgical repair of diaphragmatic hernia via thoracotomy?
a) Open
b) Percutaneous\
c) Percutaneous Endoscopic
d) External

147. What procedure does CPT code 31628 represent?
a) Diagnostic bronchoscopy
b) Bronchoscopy with brushing
c) Bronchoscopy with biopsy
d) Bronchoscopy with BAL

Male and Female Reproductive System Coding

148. What is the CPT code for a diagnostic hysteroscopic examination with bilateral fallopian tube cannulation?
a) 58555
b) 58561
c) 58562
d) 58563

149. A patient undergoes a radical prostatectomy for prostate cancer. What ICD-10-CM code is assigned?
a) C61
b) C79.82
c) D07.5
d) Z85.46

150. Bilateral salpingo-oophorectomy is coded in ICD-10-PCS as:
a) 0UT97ZZ
b) 0UT94ZZ
c) 0UTB7ZZ
d) 0UTC7ZZ

151. Circumcision of a newborn is coded as:
a) 54150
b) 54161
c) 54300
d) 54321

152. A diagnostic D&C is performed. What is the approach?
a) Open
b) Percutaneous
c) Via Natural or Artificial Opening
d) External

153. ICD-10-CM code N95.1 represents:

a) Postmenopausal bleeding
b) Menopausal and female climacteric states
c) Premenopausa menorragia
d) Premature menopause

154. What CPT code is reported for cystoscopy with ureteral stent placement?
a) 52332
b) 52334
c) 52353
d) 52356

Endocrine System Coding

155. What CPT code represents a total thyroidectomy?
a) 60200
b) 60240
c) 60220
d) 60252

156. Which ICD-10-CM code indicates secondary diabetes mellitus with diabetic neuropathic arthropathy?
a) E08.40
b) E09.40
c) E10.40
d) E11.40

157. Excision of adrenal gland tumor is coded in ICD-10-PCS terminology as:

a) 06TT0ZZ
b) 07TC0ZZ
c) 07TP0ZZ
d) 07TQ0ZZ

158. Fine needle aspiration biopsy of thyroid is reported with CPT code:
a) 10021
b) 10004
c) 10022
d) 60100

159. Hyperparathyroidism, unspecified, maps to ICD-10-CM code:
a) E20.9
b) E21.0
c) E21.3
d) E89.2

160. Partial pancreatectomy is classified under which body system in ICD-10-PCS?
a) Endocrine
b) Hepatobiliary
c) Lower GI
d) Stomach

161. Radioactive iodine ablation of thyroid remnant is coded as:
a) 79101
b) 79200
c) 79400
d) 79401

Lymphatic, Hemic, and

Immune Systems Coding

162. Splenectomy performed laparoscopically is coded as:
a) 38100\
b) 38101
c) 38115
d) 38120

163. Acute exacerbation of chronic lymphocytic leukemia is represented by ICD-10-CM code:
a) C91.10
b) C91.12
c) C83.32
d) D47.Z1

164. Injection of subcutaneous immunoglobulin is coded as:
a) 96372
b) 90384\
c) 90379
d) 96365

165. Bone marrow biopsy of the iliac crest equates to CPT code:
a) 38220
b) 38221
c) 38232
d) 38230

166. Splenomegaly is classified as a disorder of the:
a) Digestive system
b) Hepatobiliary system

c) Lymphatic system
d) Endocrine system

167. What ICD-10-PCS code indicates autologous bone marrow transplant?
a) 30233N1
b) 30243N1
c) 30263N1
d) 302H3N1

168. Therapeutic leukapheresis is reported with CPT code:
a) 36450
b) 36511
c) 36512
d) 36516

Correct Answers Test 1:

1. B
2. B
3. B
4. B
5. D
6. B
7. A
8. B
9. A
10. C
11. B
12. D
13. B
14. C
15. B
16. A
17. C
18. B
19. D
20. B
21. C

22. B
23. A
24. B
25. B
26. A
27. C
28. C
29. C
30. B
31. B
32. C
33. A
34. C
35. C
36. C
37. D
38. D
39. A
40. A
41. B
42. D
43. D
44. A
45. C
46. C
47. B
48. B
49. C
50. A
51. B
52. D
53. B
54. A
55. D
56. C
57. C
58. B
59. B
60. A
61. C
62. D
63. B
64. A
65. A
66. C

67. A
68. D
69. A
70. C
71. B
72. C
73. C
74. B
75. D
76. C
77. D
78. B
79. C
80. A
81. B
82. B
83. C
84. C
85. B
86. D
87. C
88. B
89. B
90. B
91. C
92. C
93. D
94. B
95. B
96. D
97. B
98. C
99. D
100. D
101. A
102. D
103. C
104. D
105. C
106. C
107. B
108. A
109. B
110. C
111. C

112. C
113. C
114. A
115. D
116. C
117. A
118. D
119. A
120. B
121. A
122. B
123. C
124. A
125. B
126. C
127. B
128. B
129. B
130. B
131. B
132. C
133. D
134. D
135. C
136. B
137. C
138. C
139. D
140. B
141. C
142. B
143. B
144. C
145. D
146. A
147. C
148. C
149. D
150. C
151. B
152. C
153. C
154. B
155. C
156. B

157. B
158. C
159. B
160. A
161. D
162. C
163. D
164. C
165. C
166. C
167. B
168. C

Full-length Test 2

Medical Terminology and Anatomy

1. What does the suffix -itis mean?
a) Enlargement
b) Inflammation
c) Tumor
d) Fracture

2. Which term refers to the shoulder joint?
a) Coxal
b) Glenohumeral
c) Olecranon
d) Scapula

3. Which gland secretes hormones that regulate glucose levels?
a) Pineal
b) Pituitary
c) Thyroid
d) Pancreas

4. A bronchoscope is used to examine which bodily system?
a) Cardiovascular
b) Respiratory
c) Digestive
d) Nervous

5. The prefix tachy- refers to which of the following?
a) Slow
b) Large
c) Fast
d) Small

6. The SA node is located in which area of the heart?
a) Ventricle
b) Atrium
c) Aorta
d) Pulmonary artery

7. What is the term for the outer layer of skin?
a) Dermis
b) Epidermis
c) Follicle
d) Pore

ICD-10-CM Coding Guidelines

8. What is the correct sequencing for a patient admitted with anemia due to gastric

91

bleeding from a duodenal ulcer?
a) Gastric ulcer, anemia
b) Anemia, gastric ulcer\
c) Gastric ulcer, duodenal ulcer, anemia
d) Duodenal ulcer, gastric bleeding, anemia

9. A patient is diagnosed with stage III non-small cell lung cancer. According to ICD-10-CM guidelines, how should this neoplasm be classified?
a) Acute
b) Chronic
c) In remission
d) In relapse

10. Which guideline states that codes designated with a dagger symbol should not be used as first-listed diagnoses?
a) Signs & symptoms
b) Injuries
c) Combination codes
d) Laterality

11. What is the criteria for assigning a pressure ulcer stage code?
a) Tissue layers affected
b) Dimensions of ulcer
c) Severity
d) Healing status

12. Per coding guidelines, when a condition is described as both acute and chronic, which timeframe takes priority?
a) Acute
b) Chronic
c) Current encounter
d) It is not defined

13. A patient has a diagnosis of type 1 diabetes mellitus. Which complication code may be assigned even if not documented as a current complication?
a) Diabetic amyotrophy
b) Diabetic cataract
c) Diabetic gastroparesis
d) Diabetic nephropathy

14. Probable, suspected, and rule out diagnoses should be coded as though confirmed when documented as such by the provider.
a) True
b) False

ICD-10-CM Coding
15. Which code identifies acute viral hepatitis C without hepatic coma?
a) B17.10

b) B18.2
c) B19.20
d) B19.9

16. A patient is treated for an infected right foot ulcer due to diabetes mellitus. What is the correct code?
a) E08.621
b) E09.52
c) E11.621
d) E13.621

17. Which code identifies a nondisplaced fracture of the right radial styloid process?
a) S52.501B
b) S52.521B
c) S52.531B
d) S52.541B

18. A patient underwent excision of a malignant neoplasm of the descending colon. What histology code should be assigned?
a) C18.7
b) C78.5
c) C18.6
d) C26.0

19. Which code indicates acute viral pharyngitis, unspecified?
a) J02.8
b) J02.9
c) J03.90
d) J06.9

20. An infant is admitted with neonatal jaundice due to ABO isoimmunization. What is the appropriate code?
a) P55.1
b) P58.0
c) P58.1
d) P59.0

21. A patient fell and sustained a closed pelvic fracture. What is the correct 7th character?
a) A
b) B
c) C
d) D

CPT Coding Guidelines

22. What must be documented to report an add-on CPT code?
a) Operative note
b) Medical necessity
c) Related parent procedure
d) Increased complexity

23. Telehealth services are reported with the regular CPT procedure code and what modifier?
a) GT
b) 32
c) 95
d) TU

24. Category I CPT vaccine/immunization codes report the administration and:
a) Cost of vaccine
b) Diagnosis
c) Number of doses
d) Prescription

25. According to guidelines, visceral and parietal layer closure during open abdominal procedures is considered:
a) Bundled
b) Distinct procedural services
c) Repairs
d) Incidental

26. Which modifier indicates a procedure was performed bilaterally during the same operative session?
a) -50
b) -LT
c) -RT
d) -59

27. A colonoscopy with biopsy is performed. Per CPT, the biopsy codes are reported:
a) Separately
b) With modifier 59\
c) Only once
d) Only if malignancy

28. Extensive debridement of a pressure ulcer is coded based on the:

a) Muscle layers removed
b) Wound dimensions
c) Debrided tissue type
d) Encounter time

CPT Coding

29. Which CPT code is reported for surgical resection of a malignant colon tumor?
a) 44140
b) 44160
c) 44204
d) 44205

30. A patient undergoes insertion of a tunneled internal jugular hemodialysis catheter. What is the correct CPT code?
a) 36557
b) 36568
c) 36569
d) 36570

31. Which code represents the total laparoscopic hysterectomy with bilateral salpingo-oophorectomy?
a) 58150
b) 58541
c) 58570
d) 58571

32. A biopsy of the cervix is performed. What is the appropriate CPT code?
a) 57460

b) 57500
c) 57452
d) 57520

33. What CPT code is reported for surgical debridement of a traumatic skin wound?
a) 11042
b) 11043
c) 11044
d) 11045

34. A patient undergoes bronchoscopy with biopsy of lung lesion. Which is the accurate coding?
a) 31628, 59025
b) 31622, 59025
c) 31625, 59025
d) 31625

35. Which CPT code represents a low complexity new patient office consultation?
a) 99201
b) 99202
c) 99203
d) 99204

HCPCS Coding
36. What type of temporary national HCPCS codes start with the letter Q?
a) Brachytherapy sources
b) Injectable drugs
c) Oral anticancer drugs
d) New technologies

37. HCPCS Level II modifiers are used to report:
a) Anesthesia services
b) Bilateral procedures
c) Details specific to HCPCS codes
d) Reimbursement reductions

38. A patient received an infusion of 50 mg of infliximab. How is this reported?
a) 96999
b) J1745 x 1 unit
c) J1745 x 50 units
d) J1745

39. Which HCPCS code represents a standard power wheelchair?
a) K0813
b) K0814
c) K0815
d) K0816

40. Which modifier indicates rental equipment?
a) RR
b) NU
c) MS
d) UE

41. What HCPCS code is assigned for a patient's first chemotherapy administration?
a) 96409
b) 96411
c) 96413
d) 96521

42. Category III CPT codes may be reported with HCPCS Level II codes when appropriate.
a) True
b) False

Modifiers
43. What modifier is used when one eyelid is treated during an ophthalmologic procedure?
a) E1
b) E3
c) FA
d) LT

44. A breast biopsy procedure is performed on the right side. Which modifier should be appended?
a) 50
b) LT
c) RC
d) RT

45. Which modifier indicates that an assistant surgeon participated in the procedure?
a) 80
b) 81
c) 82
d) AS

46. When a procedure is discontinued due to a life-threatening complication, which

modifier should be used?
a) 52
b) 53
c) 73
d) 74

47. Modifier -59 may be used to bypass an NCCI edit if the procedures are:
a) Performed on separate organs
b) Distinct and separate
c) Bilateral
d) Repairs

48. What modifier indicates the surgical procedure was performed only on the stomach?
a) SG
b) SU
c) ST
d) SE

49. The TC modifier is used to bill for:
a) Technical component
b) Telephone calls
c) Team conferences
d) Translation services

Anesthesia Coding

50. Which physical status modifier represents an unstable patient with an active condition?
a) P2

b) P3
c) P4
d) P5

51. When a patient is undergoing anesthesia, the anesthesia time ends when:
a) The surgeon finishes the procedure
b) The patient goes to recovery
c) The anesthesiologist is no longer attending to the patient
d) The patient is transferred to the ICU

52. An anesthesia service is personally performed by the anesthesiologist for the entire case. What modifier is reported?
a) 23
b) 47
c) AA
d) QK

53. What CPT code represents each additional 15 minutes of anesthesia time beyond an initial 90 minutes?
a) 01999
b) 01992
c) 01996
d) 01995

54. Which anesthesia modifier indicates a physical status change due to the procedure?
a) P3

b) P4
c) P5
d) P6

55. When a patient stops breathing during general anesthesia, which CPT code is reported?
a) 99100
b) 99116
c) 99135
d) 99140

56. What basic anesthesia code represents the first 30 minutes for a patient age 12?
a) 00140
b) 00150
c) 00210
d) 00310

E/M Coding

57. What constitutes the Review of Systems (ROS) in E/M services?
a) System-related questions asked by physician
b) Patient responses to system review questions\
c) Full 14-system exam
d) Organ systems related to chief complaint

58. How many unique diagnoses/treatment options must be considered to qualify medical decision

making as moderate complexity?
a) 1
b) 2 or 3
c) 4 or more
d) 5 or more

59. What is the difference between a new and established patient?
a) Complexity of chief complaint
b) Date of initial encounter\
c) Number of prior visits
d) Patient diagnosis

60. Which types of history can be counted towards E/M history requirements?
a) Chief complaint only
b) Review of systems only
c) Past medical, family, social history
d) Any elements documented

61. Physical exam levels for office/outpatient visits are based on:
a) Bullets met per system
b) Number of systems examined
c) Medical necessity
d) Time spent examining patient

62. Which modifier indicates an

insignificant or trivial problem was also addressed?
a) 21
b) 24
c) 25
d) 57

63. What code represents a high MDM new patient office consultation?
a) 99241
b) 99242
c) 99243
d) 99244

Radiology Coding

64. Which modifier indicates an x-ray service was performed for a screening mammogram?
a) LD
b) SL
c) SM
d) TG

65. A patient undergoes an MRI of the lumbar spine without contrast. What CPT code should be reported?
a) 72141
b) 72146
c) 72148
d) 72158

66. To report fluoroscopic guidance during a procedure, the time should be documented in:

a) 5 minute increments
b) 15 minute increments
c) 30 minute increments
d) 1 hour increments

67. Which of the following must be documented to code for an ultrasound exam?
a) Number of images taken
b) Probe frequency used
c) Whether doppler was utilized
d) Exam time

68. A chest x-ray is performed as two views. What is the correct CPT code?
a) 71010
b) 71015
c) 71020
d) 71030

69. The professional component of diagnostic imaging includes:
a) Technologist services
b) Equipment costs
c) Radiologist interpretation
d) Image post-processing

70. Category III CPT codes are used to report:
a) Bundled services

b) Temporary procedures
c) Routine exams
d) Permanent codes

Pathology and Laboratory Coding

71. What CPT code represents a blood count with automated differential WBC?
a) 85025
b) 85027
c) 85060
d) 85007

72. A basic metabolic panel includes all EXCEPT:
a) Calcium
b) Carbon dioxide
c) Chloride
d) Sodium

73. When coding a surgical pathology gross and microscopic exam, which modifier is reported?
a) 47
b) 59
c) 91
d) TC

74. What code represents a vaginal pap smear screening?
a) 88141
b) 88142
c) 88143
d) 88147

75. To report a timed therapeutic drug assay, the time must be documented in:
a) 15 minute increments
b) 30 minute increments\
c) 1 hour increments
d) No time requirements

76. A liver biopsy is performed. Which CPT code should be reported?
a) 88104
b) 88305
c) 88307
d) 88309

77. HDL cholesterol testing is represented by which CPT code?
a) 82465
b) 83718
c) 84478
d) 85384

Medicine Coding

78. Which ICD-10 code represents type 2 diabetes mellitus with diabetic neuropathy?
a) E08.40
b) E09.40
c) E10.40
d) E11.40

79. A patient is admitted for chemotherapy for breast cancer. What is the principal diagnosis?

a) Z51.11
b) C50.911
c) D05.90
d) Z85.3

80. Which ICD-10 code indicates a displaced closed fracture of the proximal humerus?
a) S42.201A
b) S42.202A
c) S42.209A
d) S42.291A

81. A patient underwent incision and drainage of a large abscess on the left buttock. What is the procedure code?
a) 10060
b) 10061
c) 10140
d) 11005

82. Chronic gingivitis is classified to which ICD-10 code?
a) K05.00
b) K05.01
c) K05.10
d) K05.11

83. Benign essential hypertension is represented by which ICD-10 code?
a) I10
b) I11.9
c) I12.9
d) I13.10

84. Which diagnosis code indicates acquired

absence of the right kidney?
a) Z90.5
b) N28.1
c) Z90.6
d) Q60.5

Surgery Coding

85. What is the CPT code for a total abdominal colectomy?
a) 44140
b) 44141\
c) 44143
d) 44144

86. A pediatric patient undergoes an adenoidectomy. Which CPT code should be reported?
a) 42830
b) 42831
c) 42835
d) 42836

87. Which CPT code represents a lumbar laminectomy with facetectomy?
a) 63030
b) 63035
c) 63040
d) 63043

88. What code is reported for the surgical reconstruction of a breast with implant?
a) 19340
b) 19342
c) 19357
d) 19361

89. A laparoscopic gallbladder removal converted to an open procedure is coded as:
a) 47600 only
b) 47605 only
c) 47600, 47605
d) 47605, 47600

90. Which ICD-10-PCS code indicates excision of the gallbladder?
a) 0FB40ZX\
b) 0FB44ZX
c) 0FT40ZZ
d) 0FT44ZZ

91. Release of carpal tunnel is represented by which CPT code?
a) 25107
b) 25109
c) 25111
d) 25115

Inpatient Hospital Coding

92. What is the POA indicator used for conditions that arise during the inpatient stay?
a) N
b) U
c) W
d) Y

93. A patient is admitted for acute renal failure. Chronic kidney disease is also documented. What is the principal diagnosis?

a) Acute renal failure
b) Chronic kidney disease
c) Both equally important
d) More info needed to determine principal

94. When assigning inpatient diagnosis codes, which condition is sequenced first?
a) Reason for admission
b) Most severe
c) Most resources used
d) Unresolved from prior admission

95. A patient has a PTCA of two coronary arteries with stent placement. What is the ICD-10-PCS code?
a) 02703DZ\
b) 02703D3
c) 02703D3, 02703D3
d) 02703DZ, 02703DZ

96. Initial encounter for open fracture of right radius shaft is coded as:
a) S52.321A
b) S52.321B
c) S52.321D
d) S52.321G

97. What is the ICD-10-PCS code for IV infusion of vitamin K?
a) 30233H1
b) 30233M1
c) 3E033GC
d) 3E033VC

98. A CABG using arterial graft is represented by which PCS code?
a) 0210093
b) 02100A3
c) 02100J3
d) 02100K3

HIPAA Compliance

99. What does HIPAA stand for?
a) Health Information Patient and Accountability Act
b) Health Insurance Portability and Accountability Act
c) Healthcare Information Protection and Authentication Act
d) Hospital Inpatient Privacy and Accessibility Act

100. Which of the following are examples of protected health information under HIPAA?
a) Patient address
b) Test results
c) Treatment notes
d) All of the above

101. HIPAA gives patients the right to:
a) Restrict who can access their PHI
b) Obtain a copy of their medical records
c) Request corrections to their PHI
d) All of the above

102. Under HIPAA, authorization from the patient is required for which of the following?
a) Treatment purposes
b) Billing and payment
c) Marketing communications
d) Public health activities

103. A HIPAA violation occurs when PHI is accessed without proper authorization.
a) True
b) False

104. HIPAA requires covered entities to have safeguards in place for:
a) Technical security
b) Physical security
c) Administrative procedures
d) All of the above

105. What is the penalty range per violation for non-compliance with HIPAA regulations?
a) $100 to $50,000
b) $500 to $100,000
c) $10,000 to $1.5 million
d) $50,000 to $1.5 million

Reimbursement and Billing Procedures

106. What form is used by physicians and suppliers to submit claims to Medicare?
a) CMS 1500
b) UB-04
c) CMS 1450
d) ADA 2012

107. An assistant surgeon should be reimbursed at what percentage of the surgeon's fee?
a) 50%
b) 80%
c) 100%
d) 125%

108. Which of the following requires prior authorization from insurers?
a) Office visits
b) Lab tests
c) Surgeries
d) Immunizations

109. What is the timely filing deadline for Medicare claims submission?
a) 30 days from date of service
b) 60 days from date of discharge
c) 90 days from date of service
d) 1 year from date of service

110. Medical necessity for reimbursement means the service is:
a) Ordered by a physician
b) Performed per protocol
c) Appropriate for diagnosis
d) Rule out criteria met

111. An appeal submitted to Medicare after a reconsideration denial is called:
a) Redetermination
b) Administrative law judge hearing
c) Settlement conference
d) Second level review

112. Bundling edits prevent separate payment for services when:
a) Provided by different specialties
b) Performed on different body sites
c) Considered part of a more comprehensive code
d) Delivered in multiple sessions

Ophthalmology and Otorhinolaryngology Coding

113. What CPT code represents an extensive ophthalmological exam of a new patient?
a) 92002
b) 92004
c) 92012
d) 92014

114. Excision of benign lesion of right ear auricle is coded to CPT _____ with modifier -RT.
a) 69300
b) 69100
c) 69990
d) 69799

115. Which ICD-10 code indicates acute suppurative otitis media without spontaneous rupture of ear drum?
a) H65.20
b) H66.001
c) H66.002
d) H66.4X1

116. A patient undergoes canaloplasty of the left lacrimal canal. What is the CPT code?
a) 68761
b) 68801
c) 68810
d) 68811

117. What procedure does CPT code 69714 represent?
a) Myringoplasty
b) Ossiculoplasty
c) Mastoidectomy
d) Tympanostomy

118. ICD-10 code H02.881 indicates:
a) Ectropion of right eyelid
b) Blepharospasm
c) Enophthalmos due to atrophy of orbital tissue
d) Retained foreign body in right lacrimal duct

119. Which ICD-10 code represents acquired absence of the left eye?
a) Z89.411
b) Z90.01
c) Z90.02
d) Z90.09

Cardiovascular System Coding

120. What is the ICD-10-CM code for hypertensive heart disease with heart failure?
a) I11.0
b) I50.1
c) I50.9
d) I51.9

121. A patient presents with chest pain and is found to have an acute myocardial infarction of the lateral wall. What ICD-10-CM code is assigned?
a) I21.01
b) I21.02
c) I21.09
d) I21.19

122. What CPT code is reported for insertion of a pacemaker pulse generator?
a) 33208
b) 33212\
c) 33213
d) 33249

123. A patient undergoes an aortic valvuloplasty. What is the root operation?
a) Restriction
b) Dilation
c) Excision
d) Transplantation

124. What ICD-10-PCS code indicates percutaneous transluminal coronary angioplasty (PTCA) of a coronary artery using a drug-eluting stent?
a) 027Q3ZZ
b) 027Q4ZZ
c) 02703E3
d) 02703F3

125. Varicose veins of the left lower extremity with inflammation is coded as:
a) I83.811
b) I83.013
c) I83.103
d) I87.2

126. Aortic valve disorder is represented by ICD-10-CM code:
a) I35.0
b) I35.1
c) I35.2
d) I35.9

Gastroenterology Coding

127. What CPT code represents endoscopic ultrasound of the esophagus, stomach, and/or duodenum?
a) 43200
b) 43180
c) 43231
d) 43237

128. A patient with cirrhosis of the liver undergoes a paracentesis procedure. What CPT code is reported?
a) 49082
b) 49083
c) 49084
d) 49422

129. GERD with esophagitis is represented by ICD-10-CM code:
a) K21.0
b) K21.9
c) K44.9
d) K92.2

130. What ICD-10-PCS code indicates laparoscopic cholecystectomy?
a) 0F5J4ZZ
b) 0FB44ZX
c) 0FT44ZZ
d) 0FTB4ZX

131. Closure of gastrostomy is represented by root operation:
a) Restriction
b) Closure
c) Extraction
d) Detachment

132. A patient presents with right lower quadrant pain. A diagnosis of suspected appendicitis is documented. What is coded?
a) K35.80
b) K37
c) R10.831
d) R10.83

133. What CPT code represents colonoscopy with endoscopic mucosal resection?
a) 44391
b) 45380
c) 45385
d) 45388

Neurology and Psychiatry Coding

134. What CPT code represents an EEG extended monitoring, 41-60 minutes?
a) 95812
b) 95813\
c) 95816
d) 95819

135. Cerebral atherosclerosis with chronic total occlusion

of right carotid artery is coded as:
a) I63.231
b) I65.21
c) I66.01
d) I66.3

136. Excision of acoustic neuroma via craniotomy is represented by CPT code:
a) 61546
b) 61575
c) 61580
d) 61600

137. ICD-10-CM code F84.0 represents diagnosis of:
a) Autistic disorder
b) Asperger's syndrome
c) Rett's syndrome
d) Childhood disintegrative disorder

138. Neuropsychological testing by physician with interpretation is reported with CPT code:
a) 96105
b) 96120
c) 96125
d) 96130

139. What is the ICD-10-PCS code for craniotomy with insertion of intracranial vascular shunt?
a) 009U3JZ\
b) 019U3JZ

c) 0W9U3JZ
d) 0W993JZ

140. Major depressive disorder, recurrent, moderate is coded as:
a) F32.1
b) F33.1
c) F34.1
d) F41.1

Respiratory System Coding

141. What is the ICD-10-CM code for chronic obstructive pulmonary disease with acute lower respiratory infection?
a) J44.0
b) J44.1
c) J44.9
d) J44.0 + J22

142. A patient undergoes rigid bronchoscopy with ablation of tumor. What CPT code is reported?
a) 31615
b) 31629
c) 31634
d) 31645

143. Lobectomy of the right upper lung lobe via robotic thoracoscopic approach is coded as:
a) 0BTL0ZZ
b) 0BTC0ZZ
c) 0BTC4Z1
d) 0BTC4Z2

144. Insertion of chest tube for drainage of pleural cavity is represented by CPT code:
a) 31500
b) 31536
c) 32035
d) 32036

145. ICD-10-CM code J98.09 indicates diagnosis of:
a) Atelectasis
b) Pulmonary collapse, unspecified
c) Respiratory failure, unspecified
d) Other specified respiratory disorders

146. What is the ICD-10-PCS approach for open excisional biopsy of lung?
a) Open
b) Percutaneous Endoscopic
c) External
d) Via Natural or Artificial Opening

147. Pulmonary rehabilitation services are reported with CPT code:
a) 94664
b) 94667
c) 94799
d) 97799

Male and Female Reproductive System Coding

148. What CPT code represents total abdominal hysterectomy with bilateral salpingo-oophorectomy?
a) 58150
b) 58152
c) 58200
d) 58260

149. Orchiectomy for testicular cancer is coded in ICD-10-PCS as:
a) 0VTJXZZ
b) 0VTG0ZZ
c) 0VTH4ZZ
d) 0VTN7ZZ

150. Circumcision of a newborn performed by a provider other than the delivering physician is coded as:
a) 54150
b) 54161
c) 54300
d) 54321

151. Excision of ovarian cysts is classified under root operation:
a) Resection
b) Excision
c) Destruction
d) Extraction

152. ICD-10-CM code N92.6 represents:

a) Irregular menstruation
b) Excessive bleeding in premenopausal period
c) Postcoital bleeding
d) Contact bleeding

153. Laparoscopic supracervical hysterectomy is coded as:
a) 58541
b) 58542
c) 58543
d) 58544

154. What is the ICD-10-CM code for prostatitis, unspecified?
a) N41.9
b) N42.9
c) N45.2
d) N49.9

Endocrine System Coding

155. Unilateral thyroid lobectomy is coded in CPT as:
a) 60200
b) 60240
c) 60120
d) 60220

156. Type 2 diabetes mellitus with diabetic nephropathy is coded as:
a) E11.21
b) E11.22
c) E13.21
d) E13.22

157. Excision of part of pancreas is classified under ICD-10-PCS root operation:
a) Resection
b) Excision
c) Destruction
d) Extraction

158. Fine needle aspiration of thyroid nodule is reported with CPT code:
a) 10021
b) 10004
c) 10022
d) 60100

159. ICD-10-CM code E03.9 indicates:
a) Hypothyroidism, unspecified
b) Hyperthyroidism, unspecified
c) Thyrotoxicosis without goiter
d) Myxedema coma

160. Injection of radioactive isotope for adrenal imaging is coded as:
a) 78012
b) 78070
c) 78075
d) A9584

161. Panhypopituitarism is represented by ICD-10-CM code:
a) E23.0
b) E22.8
c) E34.4

d) E89.3

Lymphatic, Hemic, and Immune Systems Coding

162. Bone marrow harvest from donor is coded as:
a) 38230
b) 38240
c) 38242
d) 38999

163. Non-Hodgkin lymphoma of intra-abdominal lymph nodes is coded as:
a) C85.82
b) C85.92
c) C88.0
d) C88.2

164. Therapeutic plasmapheresis is reported with CPT code:
a) 36511
b) 36512
c) 36514
d) 36516

165. Hb SS disease with acute chest syndrome is represented by ICD-10-CM code:
a) D57.02
b) D57.412
c) D57.00
d) D57.419

166. In ICD-10-PCS, allogeneic bone marrow transplant is classified under:
a) Administration
b) Transfusion
c) Transplantation
d) Drainage

167. Excision of axillary lymph node is coded as:
a) 38500
b) 38525
c) 38530
d) 38740

168. ICD-10-CM code D72.822 represents diagnosis of:
a) Eosinophilia
b) Lymphocytopenia
c) Neutropenia
d) Thrombocytopenia

Correct answers Test 2:

1. B
2. B
3. D
4. B
5. C
6. B
7. B
8. D
9. B
10. C
11. A
12. A
13. D
14. A
15. A
16. C
17. B
18. C
19. D
20. C
21. C
22. C
23. A
24. C
25. A
26. A
27. B
28. B
29. D
30. B
31. D
32. C
33. B
34. C
35. C
36. D
37. C
38. C
39. B
40. A
41. C
42. A
43. C
44. A
45. C
46. D
47. B
48. C
49. A
50. C
51. C
52. D
53. C
54. B
55. B
56. B
57. B
58. B
59. B
60. D
61. B
62. C
63. D

64. C	99. B	134. C
65. B	100. D	135. A
66. B	101. D	136. C
67. D	102. C	137. A
68. B	103. A	138. D
69. C	104. D	139. B
70. B	105. C	140. B
71. B	106. A	141. D
72. B	107. B	142. C
73. C	108. C	143. C
74. D	109. D	144. D
75. B	110. C	145. B
76. D	111. B	146. A
77. C	112. C	147. A
78. D	113. B	148. D
79. B	114. A	149. B
80. B	115. B	150. D
81. C	116. D	151. B
82. C	117. B	152. C
83. A	118. B	153. A
84. A	119. C	154. A
85. C	120. B	155. C
86. B	121. B	156. A
87. C	122. B	157. A
88. C	123. B	158. C
89. B	124. D	159. A
90. A	125. C	160. C
91. B	126. D	161. A
92. B	127. D	162. C
93. A	128. C	163. B
94. A	129. B	164. D
95. C	130. B	165. B
96. B	131. B	166. C
97. C	132. C	167. B
98. D	133. D	168. D

Bonus Video 1: CPC Q & A Example Tutorial

Bonus Video 2: Process of Elimination in CPC Exam

Bonus Flashcards: 300+ Digital Flashcards for CPC Exam

Made in the USA
Las Vegas, NV
22 October 2023